Praise for *Experiencing the Po*

"I highly recommend this book to everyone longing for healing. Experiencing the Power of Zero Balancing *gives us the gift of healing stories, showing how repressed trauma and emotions are released and people are deeply healed on all levels–physically, emotionally and spiritually."*

— **Peggy Huddleston**, Author, *Prepare for Surgery, Heal Faster: A Guide of Mind-Body Techniques*

"This compelling book is an excellent way to learn about Zero Balancing and the many ways it can help people. How could this seemingly simple process help people overcome vertigo, pain, and even the trauma of childhood abuse? How could it enhance spiritual and creative energy? How could it heal a lame horse? It seems magical but the authors and their clients make a strong case for its effectiveness. I can't wait to try it myself!"

— **Jean Kilbourne**, Ed.D; author, filmmaker, activist and inductee into the National Women's Hall of Fame, 2015

"This collection of case reports by Zero Balancing practitioners is a gold mine of information for newcomers to the field and for current practitioners. Quarry and King's compilation of case studies by Zero Balancing practitioners will lead to rigorous scientific documentation of the practice, expanding the acceptance and practice of the modality."

— **Margaret Siber**, MD

Praise for *Experiencing the Power of Zero Balancing*

"This is a remarkable book documenting the healing power and dynamic simplicity of Zero Balancing! In 25 interesting cases, we are touched by the wide range of conditions that can be helped, the knowledge held in one's hands, the importance of documenting what is possible and the gift that is offered worldwide. I recommend this book for all practitioners of subtle touch."

— **Susan Steiner**, OTR/L, CST-D, Instructor of CranioSacral Therapy and SomatoEmotional Release, Upledger Institute

"For newcomers to Zero Balancing, this book offers a wonderful way to learn about the many diverse, holistic and profound ways Zero Balancing is supporting people on their journeys to health and wholeness."

— **Patricia Walden**, Master Iyengar yoga teacher with one of two Advanced Senior Certificates awarded directly by BKS Iyengar and recipient of *Yoga Journal*'s prestigious Lifetime Contributor Award for being one of the country's most accomplished yoga teachers

"I found these case studies interesting, inspiring, varied, and educational at the same time. In addition, I was pleased to see how much Zero Balancing has opened doors for the practitioner for further exploration and insights."

— **Fritz Frederick Smith**, MD, Zero Balancing founder

Experiencing the Power of **Zero Balancing**

Case Studies of Journeys to Health and Wholeness

Collected and edited by
Veronica Quarry, MS, MSPT
and Amanda King, MA, LMT

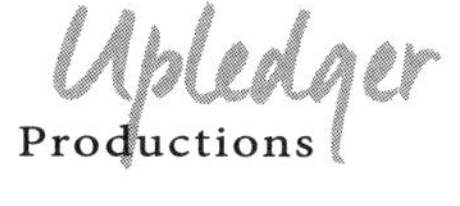

Palm Beach Gardens, FL

©2016 Zero Balancing Health Association.
All rights reserved.

The right of Veronica Quarry and Amanda King to be identified as authors of this work has been asserted by them in accordance with the Copyright, Designs and Patents Act.

No part of this publication may be reproduced, stored in a retrieval system, or transmitted in any form or by any means—electronic, mechanical, photocopying, recording or otherwise—without the prior permission of the publisher. Permissions may be sought directly from Upledger Productions Rights Department. Inquiries may be made by mail to 11211 Prosperity Farms Road, Suite D-325, Palm Beach Gardens, Florida, 33410, USA; phone at 561.622.4334; or e-mail at info@upledger.com.

LCCN: 2016935821

ISBN-13: 978-0-9907966-6-4

Upledger Productions
11211 Prosperity Farms Road, Suite D-325
Palm Beach Gardens, Florida 33410 USA
561.622.4334

Notice
Neither the publisher nor the authors assume any responsibility for any loss, injury, and/or damage to persons or property arising out of, or related to, any use of the material contained in this book. It is the responsibility of the treating practitioner, relying on independent expertise and knowledge of the patient, to determine the best treatment and method of application for the patient. –The Publisher

Editors: Veronica Quarry, MS, MSPT and Amanda King, MA, LMT
Book Design: Peter King & Company (www.king-co.com)
Cover Photos: Michael J. Williams and Todd Williams

The term Zero Balancing®, the Zero Balancing logo, and the Fulcrum logo are registered trademarks.

Upledger
Productions
Your source for educational excellence.

www.Upledger.com

Printed in the U.S.A.

This book is dedicated to
Fritz Fredrick Smith, MD,
founder of Zero Balancing,
in honor of his 85th birthday in
May 2014, and with gratitude
for his gifts to the world.

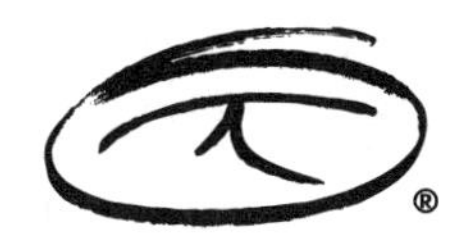

Acknowledgments

With deepest gratitude, I wish to thank my Zero Balancing mentor, Amanda Brauman King for all her time, support, encouragement, thoughtful insights, guidance and invaluable editorial assistance in helping to make this collection of ZB Case Studies a reality. I also want to thank Hadas Amiel for sharing with me her appreciation of the healing powers of ZB and for encouraging me to pursue ZB treatment and training with Jim McCormick. Through ZB sessions with Jim, I experienced relief from years of chronic low back pain (which many other modalities had not been able to relieve). I was also in awe of the increased flow, clarity and expansiveness I experienced in my chi/energy as a result of these sessions. These profound experiences led me to my own study of ZB and certification process. I wish to express my appreciation to Jim for introducing me to the power of ZB and for all his support and endorsement of this case studies project. The more I study and experience ZB as both receiver and practitioner, the more grateful I am to its founder, Fritz Fredrick Smith, MD. His work offers us a path to health, wholeness, and actualization. To all the ZB practitioners who have contributed ZB case studies for this book, I wish to express my deepest appreciation and gratitude. You have enabled my vision to become a reality and have become a model and inspiration for other practitioners to document and share their experiences.

I also want to thank the team at IAHE, Dawn Langnes and Vicki McCabe for shepherding this book to completion, and to Peter King for his thoughtful and elegant book design. Thank you.

Veronica Quarry MS, MSPT, CZB

Editor's Note

I am very grateful to Veronica Quarry for initiating the project of collecting, curating and editing these case studies on the treatment and outcomes of Zero Balancing. I was so happy to lean in to assist as her co-editor. Although I have been practicing ZB for over ten years and am well aware of its power and potential, many of these case studies left me amazed and astonished by the results of ZB in the hands of these skilled and sensitive practitioners. I would like to thank each and every contributor–ZB practitioners from the US, UK and Israel and their clients–for documenting their work and experiences so clearly and eloquently. It has been a highlight of my life to study and practice Zero Balancing. In reading and re-reading this collection, I am excited by the wide realm of healing possibilities these case studies demonstrate, and know, for each one here, there are many, many more yet to be written.

Amanda Brauman King MA, LMT, CZB

Contents

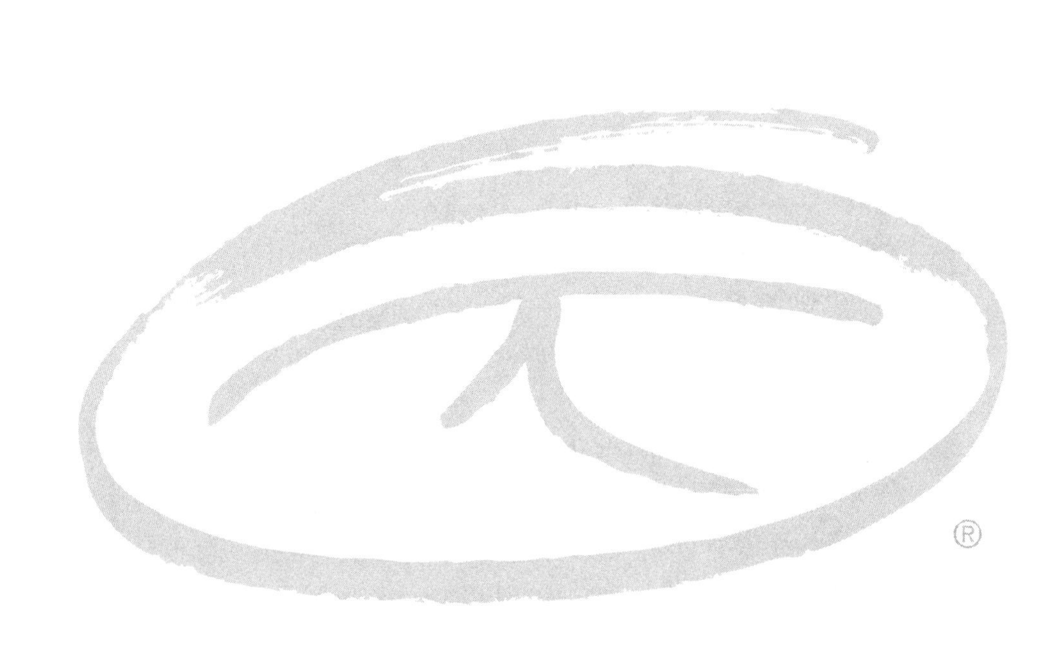

Foreword

A Message from the Founder of Zero Balancing

I have been deeply involved in the process of the creation and guidance of Zero Balancing since the early 1970s and still find it exciting to see the broad effects practitioners achieve through ZB. Our body is the template of who we are. It holds our hopes and potentials, our fears and limitations, in both our inner and outer worlds. As we alter the template the person is given a fresh opportunity for change, growth, and inner peace.

ZB focuses on balancing and clearing the underpinnings of these templates by integrating the structure and energy flows in the body with focus on the deepest tissue, the bone. These case studies show the breadth of these effects and some of the possible beneficial outcomes for the client. Reading of these experiences offers the reader glimpses of improvement of health and actualization, whether it is through ZB itself or some other natural healing form.

I found these case studies interesting, inspiring, varied and educational at the same time. In addition, I was pleased to see how much ZB has opened doors for the practitioner for further exploration and insights. I believe these case studies and the commentaries from both those performing ZB and their clients will be of interest to a large number of people–therapists and non-therapists alike–and will add to the evolution of Zero Balancing.

Congratulations to everyone for bringing these cases to our attention.

Enjoy,

Fritz Fredrick Smith, MD

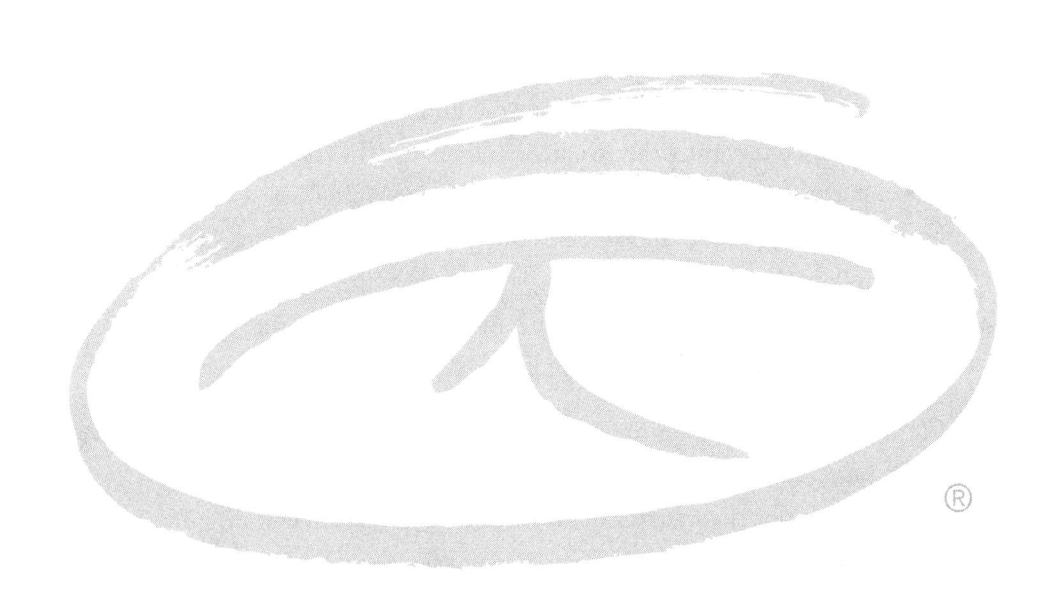

Introduction

This book is a compilation of 25 Zero Balancing case studies by certified practitioners of the modality. It is intended for practitioners of ZB and for other professionals with an interest in this work as well as clients and potential recipients of this modality.

My main goals in creating this book of Zero Balancing case studies are essentially four-fold: (1) to spread awareness and understanding of the power of ZB to promote health and wholeness to those unfamiliar with this holistic modality; (2) to establish a resource of evidence-based outcomes of ZB in order to begin a process of scientific inquiry which will demonstrate the validity and reliability of ZB; (3) to encourage ZB practitioners to continue to write and share their case studies and thus contribute to this ongoing documentation process; and (4) to offer a venue for deepening, expanding and sharing our appreciation of the power and alchemy of touch that ZB offers on our journeys to health, wholeness and awakening to our true selves.

Fritz Frederick Smith, MD and founder of ZB, wrote in his book, *The Alchemy of Touch: Moving Toward Mastery through the Lens of Zero Balancing*, the following description of ZB:

> *ZB is a hands-on body/mind therapy, which follows a protocol lasting thirty to forty-five minutes, administered to a patient horizontally reclined and comfortably but fully attired. It combines an Eastern view of energy and healing with a Western view of medicine and science. It is based on the quantum physics perspective that the particle and the wave are the two fundamental aspects that comprise our universe. In terms of the human being, I have translated this principle to signify the structure and energy of the body. Zero Balancing is a non-diagnostic system of healing. It has the stated objective to improve the balance between the structure and energy within the person's system, with the understanding that this promotes greater health and actualization.*

When we are able to receive ZB sessions, we can begin to experience the profundity of Dr. Smith's writing. A collection of case studies can also help us in our understanding and appreciation of ZB. This book describes a wide variety of client outcomes: increased range of motion, decreased pain, reversal of avascular necrosis, improved balance that had been impaired due to vertigo, relief from doubts and emotions of anger and grief, healing from childhood abuse and many other profound journeys to physical, mental, emotional and spiritual wholeness. These case studies offer us insights as to what Dr. Smith means when he says ZB "promotes greater health and actualization" of our true self.

When dealing with health care, many people want to know the validity and reliability of the modality under consideration. Case studies can begin to provide some documentation to address these questions.

In order to demonstrate the validity of ZB, we need to be able to show that ZB does what we say it does. *The Core Zero Balancing Study Guide* states that ZB is intended to provide a "holistic body therapy that amplifies a person's experience of health and vitality on all levels." Since its inception in the early 1970s, practitioners and recipients of ZB have routinely experienced the many ways that this modality enhances health and wholeness. This suggests validity of the modality but scientific inquiry requires appropriate, systematic documentation to support this. The case studies in this book are intended to offer the beginnings of a data collection process to document evidence-based outcomes of ZB and, in turn, to demonstrate its validity in promoting health and wholeness.

In order to demonstrate the reliability of ZB, we need to be able to document that this modality meets its stated goal of amplifying a person's experience of health and vitality on all levels, and that it does so with consistency and repeatability over an extended period of time. Here we turn to the basic tool that all ZB trained practitioners use: the Core ZB Protocol. The case studies presented in this book are based on sessions that were rooted in this ZB protocol and did not include other modalities. Looking at the results of these case studies, we see that the ZB protocol was effective in enhancing the health and well-being of a variety of people dealing with a wide range of physical, mental, emotional, social and spiritual concerns. These case studies also show results of the Core ZB Protocol when used by a number of different ZB trained practitioners. That this protocol can be beneficial, over and over again, to so many different people when used by a variety of practitioners, offers support regarding the reliability of ZB.

Hopefully it is clear that these case studies begin a process of documentation of evidence-based outcomes of ZB. Their contributions in demonstrating the validity and reliability of ZB are encouraging. This book is a small step in the journey of scientific inquiry into ZB, but more specific research protocols (with all the ramifications thereof) are necessary and encouraged in this process.

This book is intended to make it easy for practitioners to share these case studies with those unfamiliar with ZB. This may include potential clients, the medical community, sources of referrals as well as others unfamiliar with this modality. It is also hoped that these case studies will be a source of inspiration to ZB practitioners, potential practitioners and others interested in learning more about ZB.

It has been a joy for me to read these beautiful accounts of how ZB has affected the lives of the practitioners and recipients represented in this book. It is now my pleasure to pass these case studies on to you, to further bear witness to and share with others, the alchemy of ZB and its power through touch to promote health, wholeness and the process of awakening to our true selves.

Veronica Quarry, MS, MSPT, CZB

Editors' note: In these case studies, client names have been changed to protect their privacy.

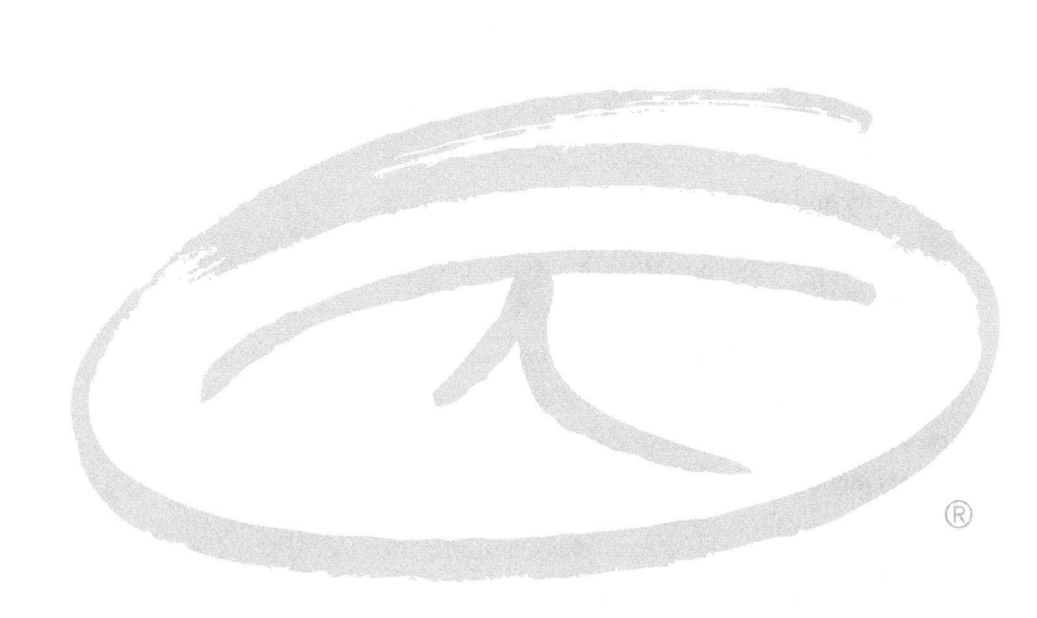

No Longer Off Balance: Zero Balancing Offers Relief from Vertigo

Elliot Abhau, BA, BS, MS, LMT, CZB

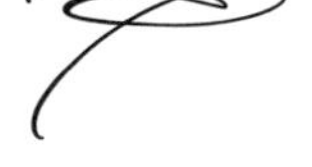

BACKGROUND

Recently I was invited by clients whose horses I treat with Zero Balancing (ZB) to attend an open house Wellness Day at a popular local saddlery in Maryland hunt country. My plan was to offer short, seated ZB sessions to the attendees. One of the saddlery's owners, Faith, stopped by my chair toward the end of the day and sat down to receive her ZB demonstration.

ZERO BALANCING

I placed four ZB fulcrums within one minute. Fulcrums are stable points created through touch, around which the body can relax and reorient. Faith then sat for a while with eyes closed. At last she opened her eyes, said thank you, took another moment, then stood up and walked back to what she was doing. Faith was certainly busy since she was in charge of the event. It appeared that her sense of duty and responsibility regarding the Wellness Day event had priority over her ZB experience and attention to her own self-care. I was just grateful that she'd asked to receive some ZB. I couldn't have been more surprised to receive the following email the very next morning.

> *Dear Elliot,*
>
> *Thank you so much for participating in the Wellness Day at our saddlery. I later realized that I was no longer off balance, literally off balance. Ever since I began experiencing vertigo a few years back, I have fallen up and down stairs, flipped over when getting dressed, banged into walls and have tipped over when talking to people. I usually spend most of my day*

thinking about staying balanced. After you worked on me, I left the store and I pretty quickly realized that I was not worrying about tipping over. I did all my barn chores today and didn't tip over! I'm not sure if it's totally gone, I still feel small effects around the edges, or that's how I can explain the feeling. So when you are up this way again, let's schedule a full session.

Thank you so much,

Faith

Practitioner: Elliot Abhau, BA, BS, MA, LMT, CZB, Horse Masters Certificate, Riding Masters Certificate, Dressage and Combined Training Judge

Modalities: Massage Therapy and Zero Balancing

ZB experience: Studying ZB since 1989, certified in 1994, ZB faculty

Location: Annapolis, MD

• • •

"Every well-placed fulcrum takes you home."

— *Fritz Frederick Smith, MD*

Acting as Witness for Tristan

Elliot Abhau, BA, BS, MS, LMT, CZB

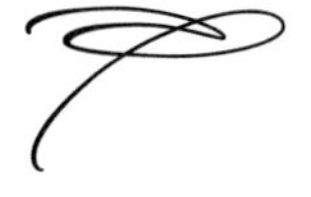

BACKGROUND

Tristan is an aged thoroughbred gelding owned by a riding school. He has a very sensitive nature. Although not suited by temperament, Tristan is expected to work as a mount for beginners, despite the fact that his right front hoof is a clubfoot. This makes him uncomfortable and skittish and therefore liable to be punished by his owners.

ZERO BALANCING

At first, all I was able to do without Tristan becoming apprehensive was simply to rest my hands on him. His coat was dry and brittle, his eyes were dull and his muscle tone rigid. He was very tender behind his shoulder blades and in his lower back. Gradually the horse responded to my touch.

Tristan's eyes, breath, and posture echoed people's experiences of ZB. These involuntary "working signs" of internal change are a means to monitor a client's process. Tristan's head lowered and his neck lengthened. His breath deepened. He shifted his weight from foot to foot adjusting his balance. Beyond this relaxation, the session did not seem significant. But when he was lead down the aisle way, the sound of his hooves on the pavement was even and regular. I could no longer hear the clubfoot and he was calm.

The stable manager reported afterward that Tristan had played in the field like a youngster and was going quietly in riding lessons. A few days later however, I heard he had become lame. Although he had never been completely sound before, he was now noticeably lame.

During my second visit Tristan was affectionate and welcomed my touch. His coat felt healthy and he was not noticeably sore. His mouth moved softly and his eyes were half closed. After the session, his walk was calm and fluid and sound!

I returned again in a week. Tristan greeted me and positioned himself under my hands. His whole right side (the side with the club foot) began to release. He started to rock and then lean into each touch. His working signs were deep and clear. The session took only 20 minutes. Tristan stood for another 15 minutes in deep process, and then became alert. He was at home in his body and in his surroundings.

Practitioner: Elliot Abhau, BA, BS, MA, LMT, CZB, Horse Masters Certificate, Riding Masters Certificate, Dressage and Combined Training Judge

Modalities: Massage Therapy and Zero Balancing

ZB experience: Studying ZB since 1989, certified in 1994, ZB faculty

Location: Annapolis, MD

• • •

"The stable manager reported afterward that Tristan had played in the field like a youngster and was going quietly in riding lessons."

Tracing Patterns of Pain

Cindy Allred-Jackson, M.Ed., CMT, CZB

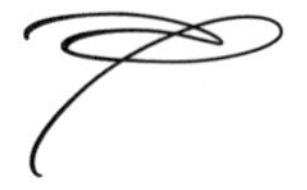

BACKGROUND

Dan is a 51-year-old, generally healthy male who travels extensively for his job. His wife referred him to me for Zero Balancing because he was experiencing sleeplessness caused by increasing pain and spasms in his left leg. During the last three years, he has used various complementary therapies that have offered some relief from his symptoms. These include Egoscue training (he continues some of the exercises somewhat regularly) and occasional relaxation massage therapy. His pain worsened six months ago and was unrelieved by epidural pain and anti-inflammatory medications administered twice by an orthopedist specializing in sciatica. Dan also unfolded details of injuries to his left leg from middle childhood through adolescence that resulted in a twisted pelvis, diagnosed in his late twenties. As an infant, he also had a cyst removed from the bottom of his spine.

ZERO BALANCING

Dan's frame (his intention) for the session was to have relief from pain.

My frame for the session was to relieve some of the cross body tension and allow him to notice and relax areas of his body that weren't painful. I knew that my basic ZB protocol would naturally address many of his specific issues. It was my job to pay attention to how he was responding so I could adjust my touch so that it felt good to him. In the first evaluation pass of the lower torso he had some borborygmi (gurgling in his stomach) that let me know he was relaxing and responding to the ZB. Working his hips, compressing the femur into the acetabulum, gave some pain relief. Slow rocking of the leg internally and externally, with one hand under the sacroiliac (SI) joint, softened the tissue and ligaments around the head of the femur. He had difficulty relaxing during the work on his feet (presumably because of old pain memories) though he wasn't currently experiencing any pain there. A particularly notable response was that a fulcrum (light pressure held stationary) into the posterior joint capsule of his right shoulder was felt in his left ankle. He got up from the ZB session standing slightly taller and felt his feet more connected to the ground.

At Dan's second session 12 days later, he recounted that the pain in his left foot had gotten worse after walking guardedly in slippery snow conditions. Relief from pain was again his frame or wish for the session. My evaluations found he had limited shoulder circumduction on both sides, the SI joint was not moving fluidly and the spine and ribs around T-10 were restricted in energetic flow and movement. During treatment of the thoracic and lumbar areas his pain disappeared for a few minutes and he enjoyed how good this felt. A few minutes later, during the normal ZB work in the upper back, fulcrums to the 8th ribs suddenly triggered pain at his left SI. I was able to diminish it some by placing the same fulcrums used early on in the session. His neck gained smoothness in motion and he showed deep relaxation with work on his shoulders and his wrists. We observed that cocking his head to the right produced more pain, and when the left lumbar area hurt, so did his left ankle. At the end of the session he had less low back pain and, after a brief period of walking, he felt lighter.

Dan's third session was four days later and he reported feeling better most of the time since his last session. "I'm feeling the love," he stated. My evaluations showed much less overall body tension. The normal protocol proceeded more quickly with several deep breaths and a few smiles. Now he was able to stay very relaxed as his feet received fulcrums. The best finding for me was that he was able to achieve an increased and smooth range of motion in his neck. When he stood after the session his demeanor was bright and he looked much taller because of his relaxed posture.

Dan has made a few follow-up appointments. He has begun to add more walking and some stretching to support his continued improvement. After six sessions, Dan has been able to return to moderate yard work and is sleeping well each night. Phone calls from his wife have verified that he is sleeping well and that he has many hours each day where he is free of pain.

Practitioner: Cindy Allred-Jackson, M.Ed. Waldorf Certification, CMT, CZB
Modalities: Zero Balancing for clients of all ages
ZB Experience: Studying ZB since 1995, certified in 2007, ZB Faculty
Location: Charlottesville, VA

• • •

"When he stood after the session his demeanor was bright and he looked much taller because of his relaxed posture."

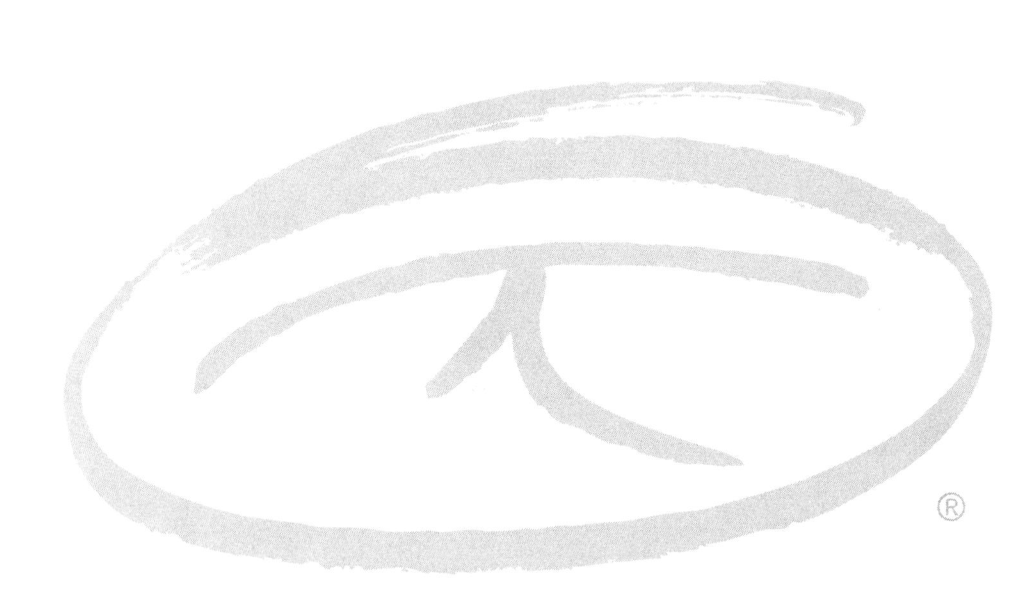

Zero Balancing and Hope: Restoring the Enjoyment of Life

Hadas L. Amiel, PT, LMT, CSLA, CZB

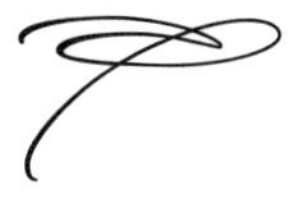

BACKGROUND

William is an 80-year-old male. Due to deterioration in his health, he moved from Louisiana to Houston to be near his daughter. William came to see me because of severe neuropathic pain in both legs and feet. He described feeling as if there were two "bars" on either side of his legs limiting his ability to walk. William also had sensory impairment and could barely feel his feet and the surfaces he was walking on. This was affecting his balance significantly.

William has suffered from back pain since his early twenties when he injured his back while lifting a heavy weight. Two years prior to coming to me, he had two back surgeries (micro discectomies at the lumbar spine, level L4-5) to address pain attributed to a diagnosis of spinal stenosis. There was no change in his symptoms following these surgeries. William was taking heavy medication for pain relief, which helped reduce the intensity of the pain, but never completely eliminated it.

William also had moderate scoliosis and kyphosis. When he came to see me he was using a cane. His back was bent forward about 45 degrees. He couldn't sit for long periods of time due to the intensity of the pain. He was also having a hard time traveling in a car since the vibrations made his pain worse.

William's normal activities had included walking his dog, watering plants and working in his garden, hosting friends and helping his wife to cook. He also liked to read. He was very upset that he could not enjoy any of these activities due to the severity of his pain–which was getting worse every day. William tried chiropractic treatment with no relief and hydrotherapy made the pain worse. Pain management doctors said they could not help him anymore. William started to lose hope that he could experience relief from his pain. Depression set in.

ZERO BALANCING

William's intention for his first session was to relax so that he could at least read.

He did not think he could lie on his back for ZB since he had not been able to be in this position for many years. He was willing to try however, so I placed a bolster under his knees and some pillows under his neck to accommodate his moderate kyphosis. I told him that we were going to limit the session to a short time and that if at any point he was not comfortable lying on his back, he should let me know and we could change his position.

On evaluation, my findings were: lack of lumbar lordosis; very stiff sacroiliac joints bilaterally, left more than right; limited internal rotation of both hips and stiffness of the lower rib cage as well as the upper back at ribs 2-9. As soon as I started the ZB session William started feeling more relaxed and comfortable. He had lots of working signs (signs that show the body is releasing held tension) that included deep involuntary breaths and rapid movement of the eyelids. He left my office feeling surprised: he was feeling less pain!

Later, William wrote:

> *My son in Maryland, studying acupuncture, suggested that his friend who is an Acupuncturist and a Zero Balancing practitioner interview me on the phone. He was convinced I could be helped with Zero Balancing. My son began a search in Houston and made an appointment with Hadas Amiel. On my first appointment, he came with me. After an interview she gave me a treatment that transformed my body. I felt as if I could fly home. That was the last time I used my cane. The pain greatly relieved*

and I was walking much better. I continued sessions twice weekly. Pain continued to decrease.

William came for his second visit a few days later and said, "I can walk without my cane. I got my legs back!" He reported that after the first visit initially he was feeling a burning pain on the left side of his leg but the "bars" that impeded his walking were gone and his whole body felt different. The following morning the burning sensation improved, too. William's intention for the session was again to relax. During the session he commented on how great the touch felt and reported that the pain and tension were leaving his body. He felt completely rested and relaxed by the end of the session and was not experiencing the burning sensation.

When William came to his third session a couple of days later he reported that he and his wife had hosted family over the weekend and that he had helped in the kitchen for a few hours. He said he paid the price later by experiencing more pain but his spirit was uplifted. He also reported reducing his pain medications, that his sinuses started to drain, and that riding in a car seemed more tolerable. His intention was to get back to feeling as good as he felt a few days ago and to be able to travel to Louisiana to visit friends for their 60th anniversary. His comment during the session was, "My whole body feels connected and alive." After working on the lower body he was comfortable with only the very small ZB pillow under his head. When he left my office he was walking much straighter and was barely noticing the pain.

On his fourth visit William said he was feeling much better and more energized. He had started gardening again, walked for an hour and that it all felt really good. He also said that sensation along the soles of his feet had improved and he was feeling his feet below him. His intention today was to improve the congestion in his sinuses. As I was working on his upper body I added fulcrums (gentle pressure that create balance points around which the body can reorganize itself) to the facial bones. William managed to lie comfortably without the need for a bolster behind his knees and with fewer pillows under his head.

I worked with William for about eight months. He continued to make improvements, became more mobile and started to walk his dog daily on foot instead of using his scooter. On occasion, he managed to travel and visit friends and family in Louisiana without much difficulty and was even able to drive himself, three hours each way, a few times. He went back to gardening, reading and enjoying his daily activities much more. His intentions became more focused on living in the moment and enjoying life once again.

Practitioner: Hadas L. Amiel, PT, LMT, CSLA, CZB
Modalities: Zero Balancing and Soul Lightening Acupressure
ZB experience: Studying ZB since 2008, certified in 2008, ZB Faculty
Location: Zichron Yaakov, Israel

• • •

"His comment during the session was, 'My whole body feels connected and alive.'"

Measuring the Effect of Zero Balancing on Standing Balance

Mary Behrens, PT, CZB

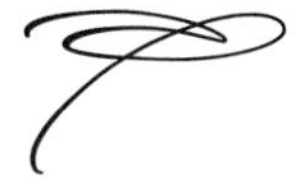

BACKGROUND

My client is a middle-aged man who works full-time in a job requiring walking over varied surfaces. A neurologist referred him to me for balance therapy.

ZERO BALANCING

This client needed convincing that this form of touch therapy would have an effect on his balance, and honestly I wasn't sure it would either! Because of his discouragement with traditional therapy, I was grateful to have something else to try with him and decided to only use ZB for our physical therapy sessions–something I had never done before.

I tested his balance using computerized posturography, a force platform in a booth that measures the client's sway under different sensory conditions and then compares the results to aged-matched norms. His results, as measured by a score well below the norm for his age, indicated that he was not using his vestibular system to maintain his balance. He told me earlier that he had a history of migraine headaches that went away when he gave up coffee, but he still experienced constant head pressure on one side. He said he often felt unsure of himself while walking up and downstairs. He depended on hand rails and was challenged in his own home when having to navigate in the dark. My assumption, based on conversations with others who work in my area of therapy, was that he was experiencing a type of vascular constriction in the area in the brain that supplies the vestibular organ, which is the organ of balance control.

Chronic migraine, if severe enough, may cause scarring to this area, causing difficulty with balance and walking in busy environments.

When establishing a ZB frame or treatment goal, the client said, "I want to feel more balanced when I walk."

The client is tall and, though not overweight, had a lot of density throughout his body. Lifting his legs for the initial half moon vector felt like lifting two tree trunks. There was so much density up into the pelvis, but he had nice working signs (visible biofeedback signs of releasing tensions and restrictions, such as deep breaths and involuntary eye movements) right away. There were plenty of dense areas to place fulcrums (gentle pressure held for a few seconds) along the skeleton and he showed many more working signs throughout.

After the first session he said the head pressure was gone, and he immediately felt steadier. For the first time since I'd seen him, he had a big smile on his face.

Over the course of ten weeks he received six or seven sessions of ZB. He also became quieter and more receptive during the duration of his therapy, softening the edge of defensiveness that he showed the first time I saw him. He expressed deep gratitude and appreciation for the ZB, and looked forward to every session.

When I retested him seven weeks later, his overall balance score had increased significantly, with near normal use of vestibular input to maintain balance. His overall score had improved to just below the norm for his age. He continued to have some ups and downs with his balance, but overall felt much more steady. He was no longer afraid at all to do the walking required for his job or to walk in his own home at night in the dark.

The progression and positive outcome for this client were a turning point for me in several ways. I am now even more confident that we are affecting many systems when we engage the skeleton in Zero Balancing.

My own understanding of a typical or migraine-associated vertigo, which was my personal diagnosis for this client, became clearer. This clarity came when, after the first session, he reported the head pressure that he'd been dealing with for years was gone. Then, an hour or so later, he said he felt more stable with his balance. I also saw how we can affect postural control in measurable ways by clearing blocks to energy flow. This is significant for me to witness as I work in a medical facility where objective measures of a client's progress are necessary to ensure the efficacy of therapy. On a different, but no less important level, the change in this client's affect was remarkable to me and very satisfying to witness. Once again, I am grateful and awestruck at the potential of this work.

Practitioner: Mary Behrens, PT, CZB
Modalities: Physical Therapy, Vestibular Rehabilitation, Zero Balancing
ZB experience: Studying ZB since 2012, certified in 2014
Location: South Bend, IN

• • •

"I am now even more confident that we are affecting many systems when we engage the skeleton in Zero Balancing."

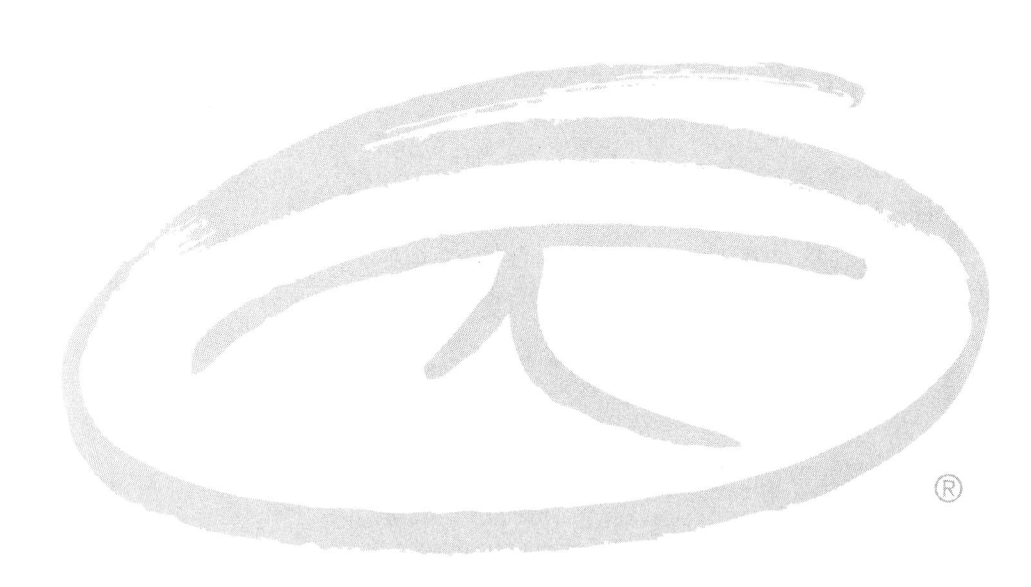

The Effects of Zero Balancing on Avascular Necrosis

Michele Doucette, BS, DC, CZB

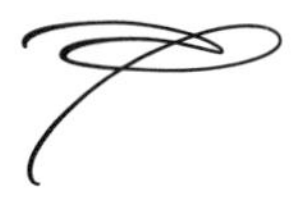

BACKGROUND

EB is a 73-year-old professor at a local university. He is a master's level, downhill mountain bike champion and former professional ballet dancer. In a local dance performance he fell and broke his hip while lifting another dancer. The fracture did not heal well and he developed avascular necrosis, a condition in which the head of the femur deteriorates and deforms, usually requiring a total hip replacement. The prevalent orthopedic thought about avascular necrosis is that in the fracture, the blood supply to the head of the femur has been disrupted causing it to become necrotic (bone death).

EB is a brilliant, active, engaging man. He had been a patient in my office many years prior to this injury and remembered the feeling of Zero Balancing and how it had helped him feel connected within himself. He returned for ZB to help him heal his femur. He was aware that avascular necrosis was considered irreversible but, with a twinkle in his eye, he told me he knew it would heal and that ZB would help. I reviewed the X-rays he brought with him which showed the typical appearance of a collapsed femoral head, a patchy, cloudy appearance to the bone, and marked degeneration of the joint space.

ZERO BALANCING

We began a series of weekly ZB sessions for about eight weeks. I also suggested he use an external electronic bone stimulator in conjunction with meditation/visualization daily, which he did after consulting his orthopedist about it. EB's intention was clear and precise: to feel the reconnection and healing of his hip. I did full 30- to 40-minute ZB sessions. I paid acute attention to his left hip using basic and advanced fulcrums, sometimes tractioning the hip and giving it space, sometimes lightly compressing and allowing it to recognize its organic self. Each session brought a new conversation with his hip, or I should say hips, since work on his uninjured right hip definitely informed his left. EB happily reported feeling energy move through his hip in each session. His range of motion and joint play progressively improved. He began to weight bear a bit more each week, but was patient and still used crutches most of the time. He reported that he just knew the treatments were helping him heal.

Within twelve weeks after beginning this series of ZB sessions he had a follow-up with his orthopedist and another X-ray was done. He brought it with him for me to review at his next ZB appointment. I was shocked to see a fairly normal looking adult male pelvis and hip. The architecture of the femoral head was almost normal, the joint space was improved, and the patchy, cloudy appearance to the bones and joint space was gone. His femoral head was alive and well! He reported that his orthopedist said she had never seen a case of avascular necrosis of the hip heal.

I commented that we may never know whether it was his own inner work, the bone stimulator, or the ZB that helped, but that it didn't matter as long as he was better. He told me, emphatically, that the ZB was what brought it all together–allowed him to FEEL the vitality return to his hip in a way the bone stimulator did not. ZB, in a way, also helped him to localize his visualization. EB was convinced that ZB was critical to his healing. He soon returned to mountain biking, dancing, and cross-country skiing.

Practitioner: Michele Doucette, BS in Biochemistry, Doctorate of Chiropractic, CZB

Modalities: Chiropractic, Zero Balancing, Nutrition

ZB experience: Studying ZB since 1996, certified in 1999, ZB mentor, ZB Faculty, co-chair Faculty Committee, chair ZB Ethics Committee

Location: Wilmington, VT

Receiving My First Zero Balancing

Karen Gabler, BA, LMT, CZB, BCTMB

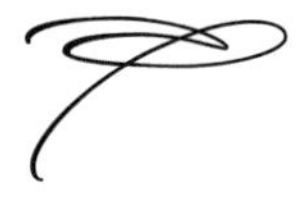

BACKGROUND

At that time in my life, I was 30, healthy, and in the midst of questioning my career as a textbook editor and processing the loss of a love relationship. I had begun seeing a Jungian therapist to help me navigate this transitional time. This therapist recommended that I see Jim McCormick at Cambridge Health Associates in Cambridge, MA for acupuncture. I followed up on the therapist's suggestion and scheduled an appointment with Jim.

I went to Jim's office, not having any idea what acupuncture was, but I trusted my therapist's recommendation. Jim took my history and did an evaluation. Instead of acupuncture, he decided to give me a Zero Balancing session.

ZERO BALANCING

My frame (intention) for the session was to be able to navigate my life changes in career and love.

I lay down on the table and Jim began the ZB session. I did not know what he was doing, but my body did. The ZB protocol begins with the lower body–the pelvis, hips, legs and feet. After Jim completed the lower body sequence, I felt distinctly how my lower body was about six inches to the left of my upper body. I saw this clearly in my mind's eye: the image of my body as two separate parts, and the lower part was in a completely different position from the upper part. Once Jim completed the upper body sequence, my whole body lined up! The disconnectedness was gone! I was aligned. I got up from that session and asked him what had just happened! Jim said he had just done a ZB session and invited me to his upcoming training.

I attended that training and so began my study of Zero Balancing, first with Jim and then with the founder, Fritz Frederick Smith, MD. I have never regretted that moment in time when the wholeness and alignment of who I am was revealed.

Practitioner: Karen Gabler, BA (Psychology/Education), LMT, CZB, BCTMB

Modalities: Structural Integration, Zero Balancing, Alignment in Movement (Gabler Sustainable Body Method)

ZB experience: Studying ZB since 1982, certified in 1983, ZB Mentor

Location: Cambridge, Melrose, Cape Cod and the Islands, MA

• • •

"Most body therapy sessions lead to a state of relaxation. When a person has experienced an essential connection, he or she experiences a response beyond relaxation–one of acceptance, internal peace and serenity." — *Fritz Frederick Smith, MD*

Zero Balancing Leading to Emotional and Spiritual Creativity

Karen Gabler, BA, LMT, CZB, BCTMB
With Testimony by Client

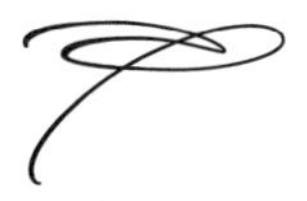

BACKGROUND

MC is 52 years old, known for his philanthropy and civic leadership. He has been receiving weekly treatments in Structural Integration and Zero Balancing with me for more than four years.

Because MC has been receiving weekly sessions over this period, we have established a deep mutual trust. Over time, MC has been able to open up and share his feelings and fears about himself, his family, and his childhood. The session described here seemed to be a culmination of that work, and was deeply felt by both the practitioner and the client.

ZERO BALANCING

The ZB session followed the typical protocol: lower body to upper body. What was unique about this session for me was that about halfway through the treatment, I began to actually see MC's bones in my mind's eye. It was as if all the soft tissue dissolved, and I was touching and working only with his bones. As I held his shoulder girdle, for example, I saw the rib cage with its individual facet joints connecting into the spine. In previous sessions, MC shared with me the fact that he was aware that he had been holding "his soldier/warrior" in this part of his body and he had been challenged to feel his own vulnerability. As I touched his rib cage, he was able to connect deeply to his soft, vulnerable side. As MC tapped down into this place of vulnerability, each of us was aware that a deep shift within him had occurred.

MC was profoundly moved by the session and went home to write about the experience in his journal. He said he felt deeply touched in a way he had not felt before. He shared the following:

> *I have received Zero Balancing treatments from Karen for several years. The serenity that the treatment offers combines with a sense of energy within my body that is delicious. That sensation of serenity and energy diminishes over the course of a few days. I often arrange my schedule so that I have the more difficult conversations I can foresee in the week as immediately after a treatment as possible. I also occasionally arrange to have the treatment just before a weekend, in order to be at leisure to savor it more fully.*
>
> *One of the most dramatic experiences I have had with Zero Balancing occurred during a treatment in the spring after I had been seeing Karen for more than four years. We had been doing some work on my shoulder girdle. It had been physically painful work, as was generally the case with that area for me. We had been talking about how much of the archetypal warrior or soldier energy had been stored there in me.*
>
> *I had always appreciated Karen and her treatments. From the first, and for years, I had been learning in these treatments a great deal about what it meant to receive: emotionally, physically and spiritually. My life as a father and a husband, a brother and a son, a leader and a follower, had been enhanced by this learning.*
>
> *In this session however, I felt a rush of emotion and sensation more profound than what I'd felt before. A confluence of grief, compassion, and communion with Karen engulfed me. I both wondered if she was feeling it, and knew she was feeling it. I have never felt so close to a person in my life, and yet it was not only Karen I was feeling close to. Everyone I knew was experienced as closer to me in this moment, and the more I*

had loved them before, the closer they had been to me, the more deeply intimate I was feeling them now. Both the confluence of these three experiences–the grief, the love, and the communion–and the intensity of each of them was new to me, and opened a space in me to experience each of them more deeply and together ever since. The result has been, among other things, an emotional and spiritual creativity I never thought to aspire to but am deeply grateful I am available to. – *MC*

Practitioner: Karen Gabler, BA (Psychology/Education), LMT, CZB, BCTMB

Modalities: Structural Integration, Zero Balancing, Alignment In Movement (Gabler Sustainable Body Method)

ZB experience: Studying ZB since 1982, certified in 1983, ZB Mentor

Location: Cambridge, Melrose, Cape Cod and the Islands, MA

• • •

"The serenity that the treatment offers combines with a sense of energy within my body that is delicious."

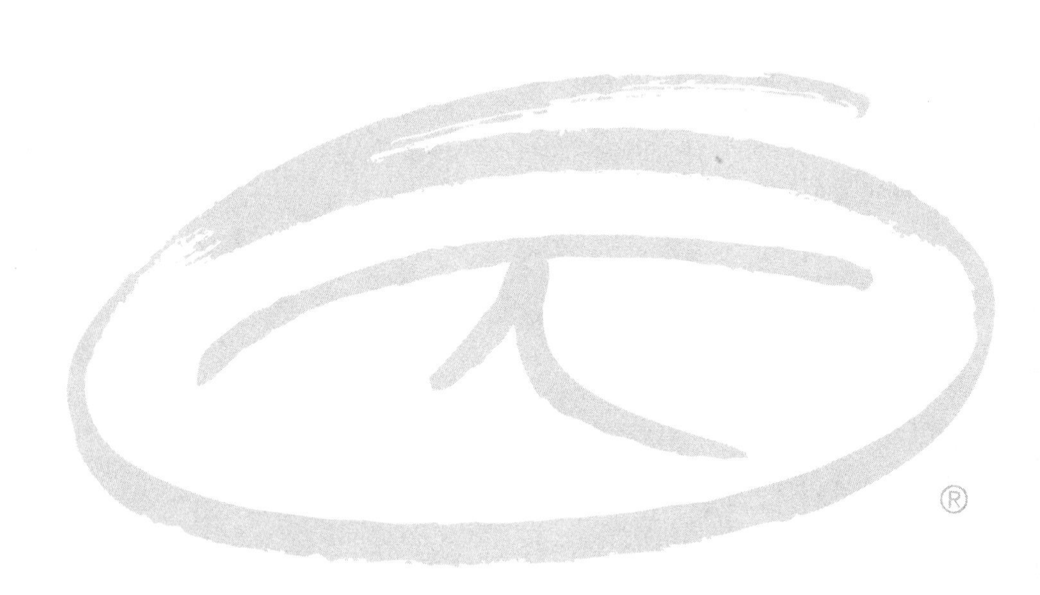

Zero Balancing for Mysterious One-Sided Body Pain

Amanda King, MA, LMT, CZB

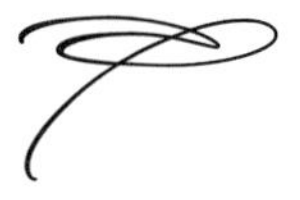

BACKGROUND

Paula, in her late thirties, worked for a major corporation in a skilled production job. She came to me originally with mysterious symptoms on the left side of her body. Specifically, she was experiencing pain, weakness, and tremors in her left shoulder, low back and hip, left arm and hand, and left ankle and foot. She described her right side as "ready to go" and her left in a state of crisis or collapse. "Both sides feel like two different people." Several months before I saw her, she had received a neurological evaluation and brain scan to rule out MS or other neurological deficit. These tests, and tests for Lyme, were normal. Before receiving Zero Balancing, Paula also received an evaluation and several sessions of physical therapy, which brought little relief from pain or weakness. Her official diagnosis was a cervical sprain, and she was seeing a physiatrist for pain management who referred her to massage therapy, which is how she found me.

ZERO BALANCING

Paula received nine 30- to 40-minute ZB sessions over the course of two months. On the first visit, Paula, who was otherwise strong and healthy, showed very little emotion. She complained of pain, weakness, tingling and tremors throughout her left side from her neck to her foot. She spoke deliberately, almost in slow motion. "I feel my whole left side is knotted up." Since the onset of these symptoms the previous summer, she was sleeping poorly and was unable to exercise because of her hip and foot pain. She felt that this contributed to weight gain and sluggishness.

I explained the flow and quality of a ZB session to her, that I would work through her clothing and first evaluate her upper back, shoulders and lower back while she sat on the table, and then I would work with her lying face up, stretching her limbs and joints, and reaching under her body, touching gently to affect the musculoskeletal system as a whole. She seemed unsure that this approach could help, since she had received physical therapy and a little massage, but was willing to try. Her goal for the session was to feel more balanced and unified right to left, and of course to reduce her pain and weakness.

On lifting Paula's legs during the first half moon vector at her feet, I felt something that I had never felt in the eleven years that I had been doing ZB. Normally, when I lift a client's legs and put in the fulcrum, I feel a flow of energy or vitality that moves up the body. Imagine lifting one end of a plastic trough of water: the water sloshes first away from you, creating a wave. Once the wave hits the far end of the trough, it returns back down to you. When I lifted Paula's legs, they felt heavy, and I perceived absolutely no movement in her energy, especially on her left side. It was like trying to achieve a flow through cement.

I continued to work on her mid-back, pelvis and hips, and gingerly on her very sensitive left foot, following the ZB protocol to address tension and balance her body. By the end of the first session, I perceived that Paula's energy began to flow. Later, she described walking better and noticed less numbness and tingling in her left hand. "The ZB is helping," she said.

By the third session she said, "I feel more balanced when I stand."

In subsequent sessions, she broke down in tears. She disclosed to me that her mother was facing a life-threatening illness and that she was her mother's primary caretaker. Other family members were also experiencing health challenges and needed full-time care themselves. It became clear that my client was holding a great deal of responsibility with little to no support, while experiencing profound grief. She was exhausted and doing her best to continue to work full-time in a demanding job, despite her pain. It dawned on me that grief can manifest in the body as a frozen energy, as the heart "sinks." The result may present as or amplify physical weakness, numbness, lack of connection, and dullness. I had seen similar body reactions in other clients after a loss of a loved one, but never to this degree. While I don't believe that grief was the sole cause of Paula's symptoms, I sensed that her emotional state may have magnified and prolonged her pain. I was glad to be able to offer her a holistic approach.

Over the course of our weekly or bi-weekly treatments, Paula was able to cry, smile and feel supported. Her back pain and left hip pain improved to the level of normal sensation. "My back is tons better," she reported. Her neck pain also improved, as did her mobility. Tremors subsided substantially. I was impressed that she began speaking up more forcefully on her own behalf. Her left foot still bothered her and she asked her doctor for an X-ray, which showed that the bones were normal. When she swapped her clogs for more supportive boots at work, her foot improved. She was pleased with the level of care that ZB was able to provide. "I didn't think this would help, but I'm a believer. ZB brought me a new awareness of my body."

Practitioner: Amanda King, MA, LMT, CZB

Modalities: Massage Therapy and Zero Balancing

ZB experience: Studying ZB since 2002, certified in 2006, ZB mentor, ZB faculty, ZBHA Board of Directors 2009-2016

Location: Salem, MA

• • •

"Over the course of our treatments, Paula was able to cry, smile and feel supported. Her back pain and left hip pain improved to the level of normal sensation."

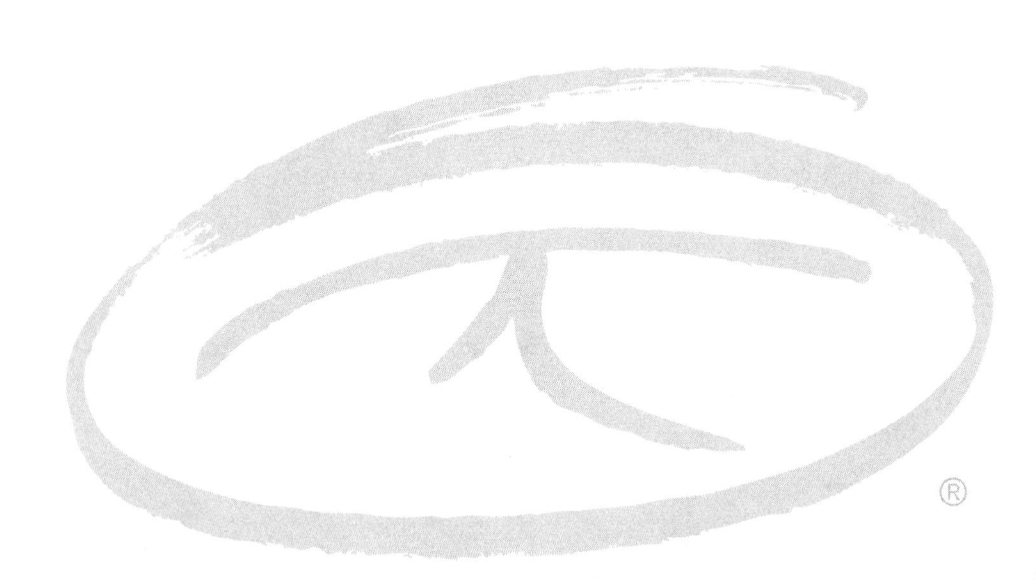

These Bones are Going to Rise Up

Athena Malloy, LMT, CBCST, CHT, CZB

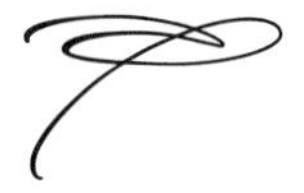

BACKGROUND

Jill is 84 years old and Sophie, her dog companion, is 15. For years, Jill saw a chiropractor who had faithfully helped her. Six months before our initial visit, he had said that she had become too frail to receive his treatments. Not only did she lose her trusted practitioner of many years, she now had an image of herself as fragile. When Jill first came for a session with me, she was bent over with mid- and low back pain. She used a cane to walk and she was having difficulty caring for Sophie.

ZERO BALANCING

The frame or intention was to relieve back pain.

After our first Zero Balancing session, Jill was surprised that she could stand up, free of pain. She was ecstatic and grateful. In the next session, she was surprised that she could comfortably lie down flat on her back, as this used to cause her great pain. As I placed fulcrums, she started singing, "These bones are going to rise up." She told me she felt I was "teaching her bones."

I had not spoken with Jill at all about what I was doing through ZB. I clearly didn't need to. She inherently understood the level at which she was receiving care. By the third session, she continued to be pain-free and she no longer needed to use her cane. She also told me about her beloved dog, Sophie, whom Jill has had to carry up and down the four flights of stairs to and from their Brooklyn apartment. Jill now brings Sophie to her appointments, and we schedule an extra fifteen minutes for Sophie to get some ZB, too.

As I apply fulcrums to Sophie's bones and joints, the energy moves more freely through her whole body. Jill says she's noticed that Sophie's lower legs are more aligned and that Sophie now easily moves up and down the stairs of her own accord.

I continue to see Jill and Sophie every four to five weeks. They are both well. In addition to Jill's frame of relieving back pain being met, she has also had a transformation in relation to her body awareness. She feels stronger and more aware of how the parts of her body are connected. She knows that how she feels physically is interconnected to how she feels mentally and emotionally.

Jill continues to write children's books and she and Sophie go everywhere together, including seeing me at my office. Jill says she feels like her bones are getting stronger. "Is this possible," she asks? I explain that as we release tension held at the level of the bone, the bones can more easily do their job of supporting the body.

Jill's zest for life is inspiring, and it has been a great pleasure to work with her and Sophie. Being a ZB practitioner is always gratifying. It has been especially rewarding to feel and see Jill become more limber and empowered in her body and her life.

Practitioner: Athena Malloy, LMT, CBCST, CHT, CZB

Modalities: Massage Therapy, Biodynamic Cranial Sacral Therapy, Reiki Master, Hypnotherapy and Zero Balancing

ZB experience: Studying ZB since 1995, certified in 1999, ZB faculty

Location: Brooklyn, NY

Reading Emotions Through the Energy Body

Jim McCormick, L.Ac., CZB

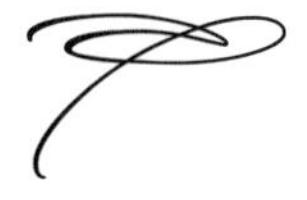

BACKGROUND

The client is a 45-year-old engineer in good health.

ZERO BALANCING

During our initial discussion, his frame emerged: "I want you to help me remove my doubt."

My client didn't specify exactly what doubt he wanted to get rid of. He was not open to doing a lot of verbal processing about it. When he stated his intention, *I* immediately felt doubt. Could I deliver on that request? Was Zero Balancing really able to help people in this way? I hadn't done this before.

I debated internally whether to accept this frame as the final goal for the session, and finally decided to go ahead, despite my reservations.

I began the session in the typical way by evaluating the body with my client sitting and what I found in his back and shoulders was unremarkable. I certainly had no clue about how to help his doubts.

However, when I went to his feet to do what we call a half moon vector (a curved pull through the legs to engage the whole body), I was astonished. I began to feel or sense energy pockets or patterns within the energy field of his overall body/mind that had a signature of doubt. The overall field had patterns like the silvery light of the moon on the sea at night. Within that field were different areas that were darker and less clear. It hit me that these were the areas of doubt. They caused me to read "doubt" like you would if you were talking to a person who was doubtful–there was a vibration particular to that emotion. As I went through the ZB protocol working with the whole body I felt many such areas.

Since this was a new experience, I wasn't completely sure, but I decided to act as if these denser, different areas were in fact where doubt was residing in his body and in his energy field. When I put fulcrums through these areas, or used my touch to create traction to pull energy through these areas, the quality of the patterns changed. The difference between these areas and other areas of the body lessened. The whole field felt smoother and more congruent and coherent, and more uniformly lit up.

By the time I finished we hadn't said a word, but I felt his system was much easier, lighter, and more integrated. He came off the table and felt lighter and clearer. He later reported that, over the next days, he continued to feel clearer and to experience less doubt.

What was most remarkable about the session was not so much this particular outcome, but the learning I experienced from doing the session. From that day forward I started to pay more and more attention to the quality of the blockages that I found in people's bodies. I learned that I could feel the vibratory signature of any emotion or any sensation in their body. Each emotion and sensation had a particular energetic signature which was unique and which I could learn to read with my hands.

If I found a place of held or blocked energy in someone's body, I began to feel more deeply–and with more curiosity–into the vibration. I paid careful attention without trying to change it. Just to be with it. I would ask myself, or ask their system, "What is the emotion or sensation being held here?" Fear had a very different vibratory quality than anger or grief. Initially I started paying attention to the major emotions (fear, grief, anger, joy) since they were the strongest and clearest, and therefore the easiest to feel. After some time, I realized any sensation that a person might be experiencing could be identified through its own unique vibration. If someone had indecision, agitation, indifference, guilt, lack of motivation and many other emotional qualities, all of these sensations showed up in that person's energetic field and could be identified through touch and then I, as practitioner, could work with them.

Sometimes this meant just continuing to do the ZB, but maybe with a different quality to my touch. If someone had fear, I might continue to work in the same places, but I might do it with a very different quality of touch. I learned that not only could I "read" an emotion in someone through my hands, I could offer an emotion with my hands. I might touch with the same quality you would use if you were to pick up a small frightened child you wanted to comfort, and hold them in such a way that they felt safe and secure. So for an adult client with fear I would do the fulcrums with that quality of touch and found that it created much greater positive change in the client. Clients with major fears calmed down, without me ever saying anything to them about their fear.

On the other hand, sometimes this opened up a whole new avenue of healing for the person. I might say to them, "I can feel a sensation in your body–I think it is fear. Are you feeling afraid?" I said this to one of my regular clients and she replied, "Only a mountain of it." This led to a huge outpouring of feeling and tears from her. We had a long conversation we'd never had before about her fears, and this led to major changes, not only for that session, but also over time. The possibility of verbally processing emotions discovered through the body/mind connection via touch opened much deeper possibilities of healing and change for people and led me to work in very different ways.

And this was but one of hundreds of such sessions where the person's experience was palpable in their body and in their field. Working with this vibration takes a person beyond help for reported symptoms alone. It can help a person connect to his or her core self and to grow personally.

So, the request that I help someone with his doubt led to major revisions in how I work and how I am able to help clients. This continues to be a major way of working–and allows the same ZB protocol to be performed in many different ways that mirrors both the physical and the emotional experience of the client, and actually helps them progress faster and deeper in their lives.

Practitioner: Jim McCormick, L.Ac., CZB

Modalities: Five Element Acupuncture, Zero Balancing

ZB experience: Studying ZB since 1974, certified in 1990, ZB faculty, past Chairman ZBHA Board of Directors, Chairman of the Board of Zero Balancing Touch Foundation

Location: Cambridge, MA

• • •

"I learned that not only could I read an emotion in someone through my hands, I could offer an emotion with my hands."

Transforming Childhood Abuse Trauma

Rosanna Price, BA, Adv.Lic.Ac., MBAcC, CZB
With Testimony by Client

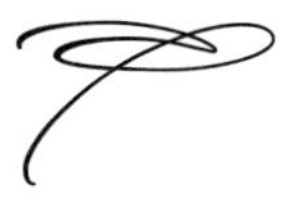

BACKGROUND

Joanne is a 50-year-old female. When she first came to me for Zero Balancing she reported feeling stressed and depressed. She was not eating properly, which in the past had led to severe anemia. She was currently on 40 mg of Citalopram for depression.

ZERO BALANCING

ZB Frame (goals for the first session): To "put last year behind me" (in which she'd been off work for three months), to normalize eating (away from eating well for a few days followed by five days of eating nothing but chocolate), and "to be able to move away from my past." This last statement was accompanied by a marked inward shift in Joanne, which led me to suspect that she was referring to a history of abuse–but, in spite of my gentle encouragement to say more, her reticence increased.

What follows is the client's own report of her experience of 35 ZB sessions, received over the course of more than a year:

> *I never thought I was heading for a life-changing experience the day I finally rang to make an appointment for Zero Balancing after carrying around Rosanna's leaflet for months. I was at a low ebb, on anti-depressants to treat the unremitting depression I'd had since early childhood. I knew medication alone wasn't going to help me make sense of my life or find meaning and purpose in it. The description of*

Zero Balancing called to me on some level, not least the fact that the recipient remained fully clothed.

Despite working confidently as a nurse for years, I really struggle when one-to-one with strangers. But from the first phone contact I knew there was going to be something different about this. I felt Rosanna was sincere, and would take me seriously. Before my first appointment I was highly stressed–I had my back-up plan of "not going" ready...and of course I only thought I would be going once anyway. That seems funny now!

Being in a strange room with a closed door raised my anxiety levels to "High Alert." I can usually conceal this, but Rosanna noticed I was clenching and unclenching my left hand. When she gently asked me about it I knew I was at a critical juncture in my life–was I going to trust this person, or was it time to run out of the room? I am so glad I stayed.

You see, I was sexually abused as a child, and my parents had a troubled relationship. My mother said I was an unwanted baby and hurt me physically at times. Fortunately, neighbors let me into their homes and fed me regularly, and I liked the positive attention I received from schoolteachers for being a good student. Throughout my childhood I was questioned about whether I was "all right," but the message drummed in to me from my parents was that outsiders should be told everything was "fine" at home–and from the abusers that "it" was a secret which would cause ME trouble, not them, if it was spoken about. Looking back–as I now can without either complete denial or total agony–I understand why it took me so long to reach out for help and why my experiences affected me and my life choices so badly. I'm writing this because, throughout the many years when I couldn't talk to anyone, I gained some comfort from reading accounts of women who had not only survived rape but were living their lives not dominated by suicidal thoughts, fear and self-loathing. Perhaps someone like me, reading this, might feel able to find a Zero Balancing practitioner and that might be life-changing for them too.

The first session is a bit of a blur but the absolute key message was that, with all my issues around being touched, I found Zero Balancing touch completely different from anything I'd experienced before. The concept of "Interface touch" (touching another with clear awareness and of physical and energetic boundaries) is amazing–it feels completely safe to me, and having never truly known this feeling before, it is the most wonderful gift.

At first I was very averse to being touched, but a great thing was that the sessions were structured to take this into account. Having explained the difference between "hurt good" and "hurt bad," Rosanna repeatedly checked in verbally with me, and also picked up on my body language, and how I was coping with the touch. It dawned on me during one particular session that she REALLY meant I was allowed to say if I didn't like something she was doing and that in itself was a redefining moment for me. There were times when I had to get up and leave the room, as I was feeling overwhelmed, and I did have flashbacks of traumatic experiences; however, unlike before, something else was happening at another level (I think I mean in my bones) and I KNEW I was getting better. I was getting in touch with a part of myself that was uncontaminated and had a real joy for living.

Over time the suicidal feelings I'd always had began to lessen their grip, and I was discovering a potent inner source of energy and empowerment. The sessions during which suicidal thoughts and urges began to leave me felt amazing in a way that it is hard to put into words–like a very strong physical sensation rushing through me and then exiting my body, leaving me feeling acutely alive and profoundly grateful to be alive. And, by facing distressing feelings during the safety of a Zero Balancing session, this meant that in my day-to-day life they were no longer affecting me so much. I realized that although the past had defined so much, it didn't have to define my future. I could put down my burdens and I no longer wanted to harm myself. I became the person that was hiding inside me all that time anyway!

It's not possible to describe every Zero Balancing session I have had, but it is true to say that I've taken something away from each one–from feelings of deep calm to recall of memories I'd forgotten, from great sadness to genuine happiness–and much more. As I grew more able to cope with touch I found I was profoundly re-connecting with life–be that nature, art, people, and my own spirit. I distinctly remember the first time Rosanna held my head. I thought for a moment that it might come apart from my body. You can see how much progress I've made! And along the way there's also been humor and enjoyment, too. Zero Balancing is a journey we've undertaken together, and I like looking back and seeing how far I have come. Discovering I could be happy is an incredible feeling that has not left me. I still have low times but I don't feel like a victim anymore. I actually like being me! —*Joanne*

Practitioner: Rosanna Price, BA, AdvLicAc., MBAcC., CZB
Modalities: Acupuncture and Zero Balancing
ZB experience: Studying ZB since 1991, certified in 1999, UK faculty member
Location: Northamptonshire, UK

• • •

"The absolute key message was that, with all my issues around being touched, I found Zero Balancing touch completely different from anything I'd experienced before."

Releasing Guilt and Transforming Relationships

Veronica Quarry, MS, MSPT, CZB
With Testimony by Client

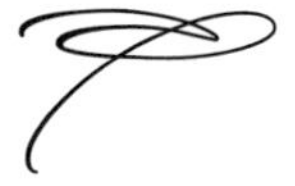

BACKGROUND

Joy and I met through mutual acquaintances. Knowing my respect for Zero Balancing, she scheduled four appointments with me over a period of nine months in order to experience this system of touch therapy. She has experienced many complementary therapies over the years, but ZB was new to her.

Joy is a relatively healthy 73-year-old woman. She continues to be very active in the visual arts. This can be physically challenging since it often involves working with large pieces of artwork. She loves to swim and enjoys walking with friends. At her first visit she reported experiencing chronic pain in her right foot, specifically the plantar region of her right heel, throughout the previous year. Walking was difficult and sometimes almost impossible because of the pain. Joy had seen many doctors but there was no clear diagnosis. On further questioning, she reported having severely injured that foot decades ago.

ZERO BALANCING

Joy's specific frame (intention) for these sessions was to reduce the pain and increase the function of her right foot. Her more global frame was to unblock or release whatever she held that was not serving her in her relationships and that did not support her spiritual journey and mission in life.

On her first ZB evaluation, Joy's passive range of motion in circumduction of her right shoulder was very restricted in the posterior/superior quadrant. (During this part of the evaluation, she reported that she had been experiencing chronic right shoulder problems.) Other significant findings in the evaluation included a very restricted right hip and sacroiliac joint; her right heel felt congested and the right tarsals were very restricted. She also held a lot of tension in her upper ribs.

Joy responded well to ZB in many ways. On re-evaluation after each session there was progressive freedom in her restricted areas. At the end of her first ZB session, Joy was independently able to circumduct her right arm and reported that she could do this with far less pain. On her third visit, Joy reported that her right shoulder has been doing extremely well since her first ZB session.

During these nine months, Joy experienced some interesting insights regarding her foot pain. She is a very compassionate and generous person, but reports a history of always needing to "come to the rescue." She thinks she frequently creates and participates in co-dependent relationships in this process. Joy reported feeling an increased clarity that part her foot "problems" are her body's way of making her slow down and inhibit her from continuing old, unhealthy patterns. Her immobility has also given her time to do things that she loves, such as focusing on her art and meditation practice. She was certain that these secondary gains were slowing her rate of recovery since she loved "having the excuse" to stay home and not be able to respond to others' needs. Nevertheless, Joy reported that each ZB session was extremely helpful both physically and emotionally. She is currently able to walk about a mile.

Regarding her more global frame, to unblock or release whatever she holds that is not serving her in her relationships and that does not support her spiritual journey and mission in life, Joy writes the following:

> *The ZB experiences I have had with Veronica Quarry have been profound and life-changing. One session connected me to my late husband who died 35 years ago. All these years I carried sadness and guilt because of hurting him. During the session I released these old feelings. I felt his love*

and forgiveness. Now I feel clear and the great sense of guilt is no longer heavy on my heart.

The other session related to my daughter. There was a lot of sadness after a falling out we had twelve years earlier. Things were never the same, and I felt a great sense of loss. During a session with Veronica, that was lifted. Veronica is a beautiful healer. I felt completely safe to let the session unfold as she worked on me in her gentle, nurturing and powerful way. My body was shaking as it released the old memories.

Since the session, the relationship with my daughter has greatly changed. I no longer have the feeling of distrust and discomfort. Our relationship is loving and comfortable. I accept her as a beautiful mother, person, talented creator and most of all a friend. I have moved into acceptance, rather than trying to fix her and her family.

Working with Veronica and experiencing Zero Balancing has truly been an amazing life-changing experience. – Joy

Practitioner: Veronica Quarry, BS, MS, MSPT, CZB
Certifications: Early Intervention Specialist, Prepare for Surgery, Heal Faster
Modalities: Physical Therapy, CranioSacral Therapy, Lymph Drainage Therapy and Zero Balancing
ZB experience: Studying ZB since 2013, certified in 2014
Location: Greater Boston

• • •

"During the session I released these old feelings. I felt his love and forgiveness."

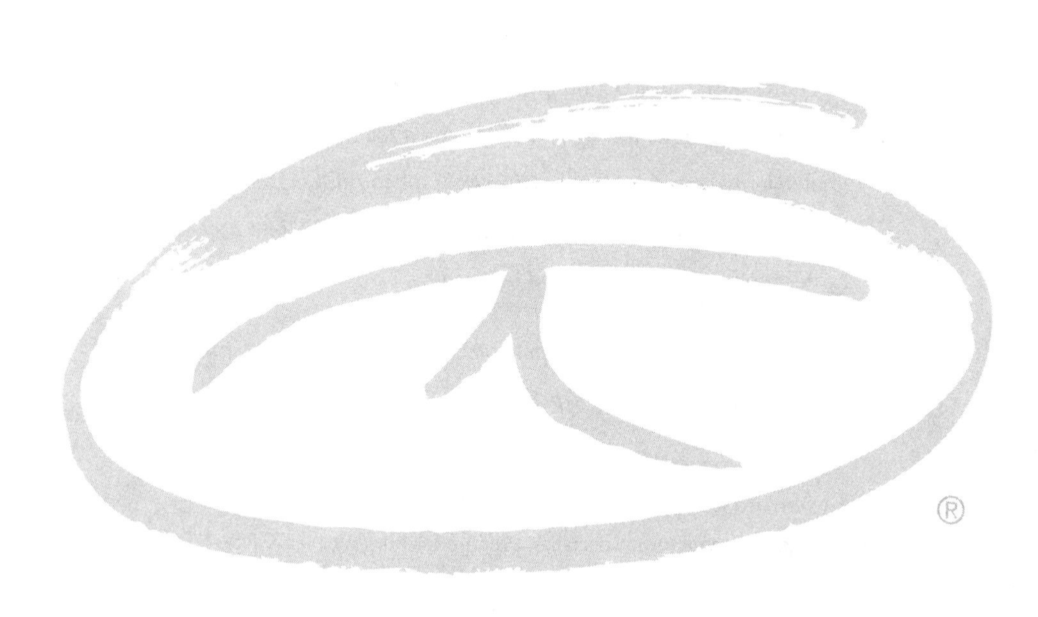

Releasing Pent-up Stress and Trauma with Surprising Results

Veronica Quarry, MS, MSPT, CZB
With Testimony by Client

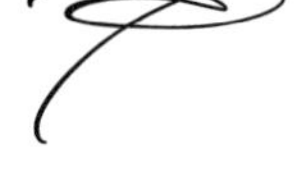

BACKGROUND

AW is a 62-year-old woman who has had a successful 25-year career in massage therapy. AW routinely engages in aerobic activities to challenge her cardiovascular system. I met AW while on a women's retreat in Rhode Island. During that time I offered the women there complimentary Zero Balancing sessions. AW was one of several who accepted my offer. The session took place in a separate room offering privacy from the other retreat attendees. The session was rooted in the Core ZB protocol, which touches the whole body from head to toe. Six months later, AW wrote the following:

> *The last twenty years of my life have been less than ideal. I had recently ended a twenty-year marriage with a verbally abusive alcoholic spouse when I met Veronica at a retreat. My health had been compromised. My husband and I had been fighting nonstop, and I felt like I had lost my ability to feel anything at all. My tears had all but dried up, and laughter had vacated the building. At the same time, I had been diagnosed with celiac disease and was also dealing with that challenge. In leaving the marriage, I had to go through bankruptcy, foreclosure and then the final trifecta, divorce. I was in a state of despair.*
>
> *I have spent my life, at least twenty-five years of it, as a massage therapist in the mountains of Colorado. I love being a healer and thought that I had experienced every modality that the healing arts had to offer.*

After participating in a weekend retreat with a women's group focused on Awakening, Veronica asked if we would like to receive a Zero Balancing session from her. I had never heard of Zero Balancing, and didn't know anything about how it works, but had great respect for Veronica. So I was thrilled for the opportunity. I had no idea what the next hour of my life was about to unfold and unwrap and unwind for me.

ZERO BALANCING

Veronica had me lie on a massage table with my clothes on and she put her hands on my feet. Her hands felt peaceful and I was expecting to drift off into a nice state of relaxation. As she moved to my pelvis and my back, within a few minutes I felt a slight quivering throughout my body, almost like I was cold, but I knew I wasn't.

The quivering quickly escalated to a mild shaking. I was a bit concerned but decided to go with the flow, as they say, and let my body do what it was naturally doing. As Veronica worked, thoughts and feelings starting flashing before my eyes and I could feel deep waves of emotions. Although not cathartic, they were powerful and moving. It was as though someone had uncorked my energetic body and energy started to release slowly but very powerfully. Then the next thing I knew I started to shake in a way that felt uncontrollable and almost violent. I could no longer keep the cork on my body's energy system; a crack had formed and release was inevitable. Fear started to come up. Sensing my concern, Veronica stopped the session and asked if I was okay. "Yes," I said, "but what is going on?" Knowing my history, she mentioned a book, Waking the Tiger: Healing Trauma *by Peter A. Levine. She said that when animals escape a predator, they shake or tremble for a while so that their bodies can release the trauma of the event. Humans, especially adults, she said often don't do that. Instead, we tend to store the trauma in our bodies and bones. To our detriment, we can drag our traumas around with us, often for our entire lifetime(s).*

We both took a few breaths and then went back to the ZB treatment, and I was now able to relax into the releasing. My body continued to shake violently for what seemed like a long time, and then sounds started to come out of my mouth that felt like an energetic exorcism of sorts. I couldn't stop them if I wanted to. It was bigger than me, and at that point it almost became pleasurable–as any deep, deep release would be.

My body and energy finally started to come to a place of rest, and I felt like I had just run a marathon: deeply tired, but euphoric and calm. When the session was over, Veronica and I talked about what had happened, and I had an amazing realization. I had experienced, for most of my grown life, what probably would have been diagnosed as Restless Leg Syndrome. I have had to shift, and move, and fidget with my legs for decades. I know they make a drug for that, but I just lived with it and never really knew why I would have such restless extremities.

Then the light went on! I was sure that I had unconsciously pushed all the traumas that had occurred in my life down into the lower part of my body where they must have been stored in my bones. In the next few months after this ZB session, my legs were no longer restless and my feet had no need to shake and fidget. I was blown away.

I am still in awe of that one-hour transformational experience that an amazing healer and teacher gifted me. How could so much pain and emotional abuse be released in such a short period of time? Willingness on my part to show up and let go, and allow Zero Balancing to be the doorway to my freedom.

It has been about six months since the session, and my life has changed in so many ways. The Restless Leg Syndrome is gone. I find myself in a much more relaxed and peaceful state much more of the time. I have opened myself up to a man in my life who treats me with respect, compassion and love. We are able to express our feelings with each other. My whole body seems to be awake and alive and I have more energy than I've had for a long, long time.

I am forever grateful to the woman who uttered the words, "Would you like to have a Zero Balancing session?" "Yes," I said. And if you ever have the opportunity to receive one for yourself, I encourage you to respond in like manner. – AW

I am deeply grateful to AW for writing about her profound first experience with Zero Balancing. It's a wonderful testimony to the alchemical nature of ZB, in its possibility to bring us into healthier states of being while supporting us in the transformational process of Self-Realization.

In ZB we typically have our clients set a "frame" or intention for each session. As a practitioner, my frame for the client (though not typically verbalized) is that the ZB will allow the client to release anything they hold that no longer serves their Highest Good. Experience has given me great confidence in this process and I was very comfortable holding sacred space for AW as she went through her releasing process. I also want to acknowledge AW's courage, confidence and maturation in her journey. As she said, it was, "willingness on my part to show up and let go, and allow Zero Balancing to be the doorway to my freedom." I trust that we show up and let go, as each of us is ready and able to do so.

– Veronica

Practitioner: Veronica Quarry, BS, MS, MSPT, CZB

Certifications: Early Intervention Specialist, Prepare for Surgery, Heal Faster

Modalities: Physical Therapy, CranioSacral Therapy, Lymph Drainage Therapy and Zero Balancing

ZB experience: Studying ZB since 2013, certified in 2014

Location: Greater Boston

• • •

"When you are in touch with motion, you are in touch with energy." — *Fritz Frederick Smith, MD*

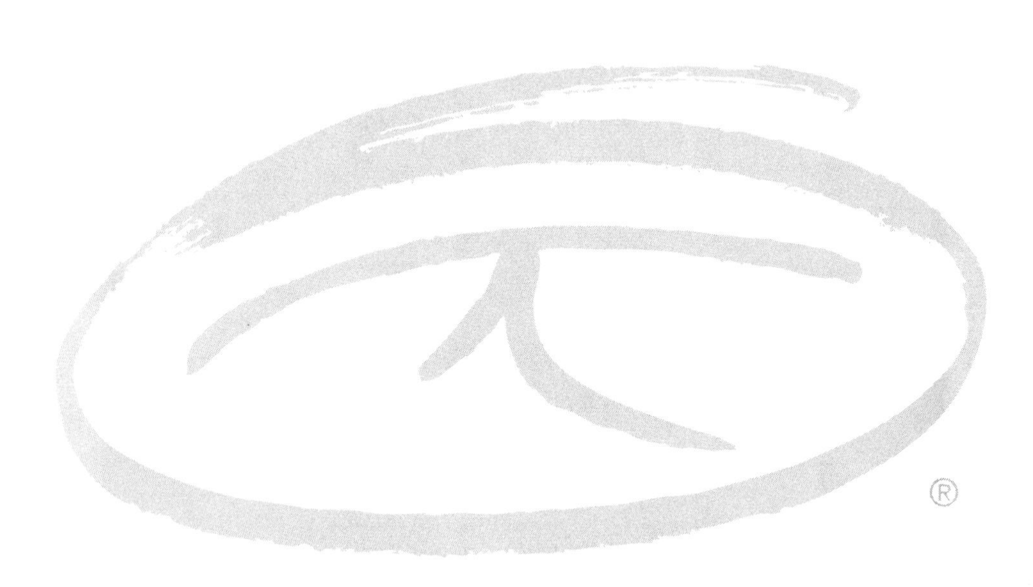

Forging the Bones of the Earth

Terry Lillian Segal, LMT, CZB

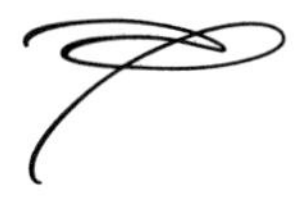

A tall, gaunt, lanky gentleman with eagle-sharp features enters my studio, speaking in slurred and labored language. He is sliding into a rapid decline from his recent diagnosis of amyotrophic lateral sclerosis (ALS), commonly referred to as Lou Gehrig's Disease. This mild-mannered man who was, until recently, a stalwart hulk of a figure, wielding huge chunks of iron, honing them into powerful works of art, now teeters like a reed in the wind. He requests my services to assist with his balance, and with his breathing.

I had the incalculable privilege of working weekly with RJ for the last two years of his life. Not long into our work together, he lost his capacity for intelligible speech, and began to communicate via an electronic talking pad that resembled the old "Etch-a-Sketch" toys to describe images, precise or garbled, as we drew mechanical lines in the sand. Such was RJ's dance with the ghoulish specter of ALS, which continually repositioned that line in the sands of RJ's tenacious, courageous journey, one grueling step at a time.

RJ loved Zero Balancing, which was the sole modality I utilized with him, and I loved sharing it with him. I could feel his life force galvanized and mobilized in his prominent skeleton–could feel the liquid accumulation in his lungs, and the quieting thereof, as the session progressed each week.

RJ and I rarely spoke, yet we communicated with incredible depth and mutual understanding. I understood that as a metalsmith, his medium of expression was through the Bones of the Earth. Mine, through the bones of our astoundingly vulnerable and strong bodies. As I considered all that went into RJ's relationship to metal, it "struck" me as notably parallel to all of the working principles of ZB. Even though he subjected the raw materials to the fires of change and worked a hard discipline into them, still, all of this was done with the intent of Interface. For just as Michelangelo experienced the emergence of his creations from the stone, RJ's creations had a similar quality of being the Essence of something invited forth, by the act of being Met, held in the fulcrum of numinous suspension in the timeless space of the Present Moment. Twice, towards the end of his remarkable life, RJ tapped out a note to me on his little talking board: that he loved ZB because it was the one thing that truly helped him to breathe, easing the tension in his rib basket, quieting his nervous system, and grounding him into his physical body.

Given that he spent much of his time vacuuming out his lungs via the long proboscis of a sucking machine beside his bed, this felt to me to be the greatest gift possible from the work.

RJ made a Herculean gesture in the last months of his life, gathering together nearly thirty pre-eminent metalsmiths to work in concert under his guidance to create a monolithic sculpture that he dedicated to his beautiful wife, who was by his side with unflagging devotion. He was finally laid down in green pastures one week after the public dedication of his work.

My association with RJ touched me deeply, and energized my ongoing awe for the exquisite power and artistry of ZB. His recommendation of my work to the local hospice agencies facilitated the extension of my practice into that tender arena, which was another life-changing turn on my Spiral, both personally and professionally. Our wordless relationship resonated down to the bone, and I shall never, ever forget him for the countless gifts he gave me, for being such an inspiring model of courage, tenacity, grace and grit, and for all that we were able to share because of the fundamental beauty of Zero Balancing.

Practitioner: Terry Lillian Segal, LMT, CZB
Modalities: Massage Therapy and Zero Balancing
ZB experiences: Studying ZB since 1993, certified in 1999, ZB mentor
Location: Cleveland Heights, OH

• • •

"I could feel his life force galvanized and mobilized in his prominent skeleton."

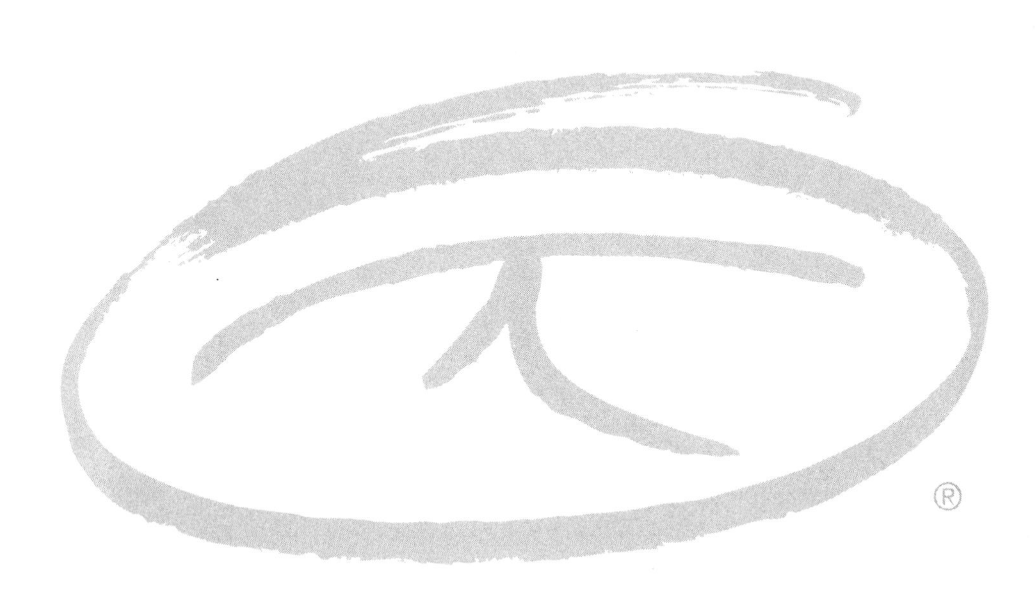

Easing and Increasing Neck Range of Motion

Maureen Staudt, BSN, RN, LMT, CZB

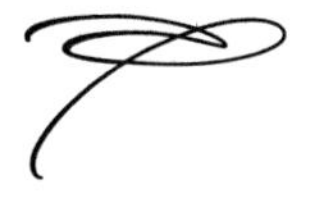

BACKGROUND

TL originally came to me for shoulder and neck achiness. She stated that she had difficulty turning her head to the right. Her level of pain on this visit was 3 out of 10 (10 being the worst). She admitted that the pain reached an 8 out of 10 at times. She said that her chiropractor often had a difficult time adjusting her neck to the right side.

ZERO BALANCING

On evaluation, TL's upper back, scapulae and shoulder girdles were very dense and tight. Her neck range of motion was sluggish on rotation to the right. I performed a 40-minute Zero Balancing session on TL. Because of the restrictions I felt in her neck, I chose to use three special neck fulcrums, which gently aim to improve flow through the full cervical spine and free upper cervical joint restrictions between C1 and the occiput and C1 and C2. On re-evaluation the client's neck moved much more easily. In fact, a tear came from her eye after the treatment when she realized how easily her neck was moving.

TL returned to see me the following week. She was amazed at the results that she received from one ZB session. She passed out my brochures to many of her friends. She admitted that she had no occipital pain since the last visit.

TL now comes once a month for a maintenance ZB session. She is very pleased at the results she gets from Zero Balancing.

Practitioner: Maureen Staudt, BSN, RN, LMT, CZB

Modalities: Zero Balancing

ZB Experience: Studying ZB since 2004, certified in 2006, ZB mentor, ZB faculty

Location: Souderton, PA

• • •

"A tear came from her eye after the treatment when she realized how easily her neck was moving."

Pain in Legs that Affects Her Sleep

Maureen Staudt, BSN, RN, LMT, CZB

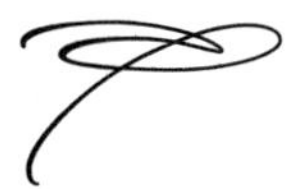

BACKGROUND

TC is a 70-year-old woman who was referred to me by one of my clients. TC came to her first visit with a complaint of chronic pain in her legs. She reported taking diuretic and blood pressure medications and experiencing arthritis pain at times throughout her body. She said she did not have other health concerns at this time and reported being fully functional in activities of daily living.

TC said the pain in her legs began a year ago after she'd had three falls on ice. Today, she rated her pain as a 6 on a scale of 0-10 (0 being no pain, 10 being the worst pain experienced). She reported seeing numerous physicians for this pain, including an orthopedist and a sports medicine doctor. Diagnostic tests included an EMG, an MRI and X-rays. She was told there was no visible reason for her pain. At one point she had been put on steroids but had to discontinue these medications because of the side effects. At this time, she was having difficulty going to sleep and staying asleep due to the pain in her legs.

ZERO BALANCING

Zero Balancing Frame: TC's intention for the session was to have less pain in her legs and be able to sleep through the night.

On evaluation, I experienced many areas throughout TC's body that were dense and tight, including her neck, arms, sacrum and right hip. Tension in her tibias and Achilles tendons were particularly noticeable, and her right ankle felt stuck and unable to move.

I did a 40-minute ZB session with TC. I added special fulcrums for her tibias and fibulas. I could feel change and movement while using these fulcrums on her legs and I placed extra fulcrums into her Achilles tendons. I could feel the tension ease in her Achilles by approximately 80%. I utilized special neck fulcrums as a result of the restrictions I found in her neck.

Numerous times during this session TC commented that she felt no pain while lying on the massage table. She verbalized that she hoped she would be able to sleep that night. I encouraged her to be kind to herself the rest of the day and to notice any little changes in her body. I also requested that I see her two more times.

I saw TC a total of three times during that first month. On her second visit she stated that she felt good for four days after her initial ZB session. She said ZB has been the only treatment to date that has given her relief from the pain. After the fourth day, she said, the pain in her legs resumed. The pain becomes worse at night and is mainly in her right hip. This time we worked for 35 minutes.

On her third visit she admitted that she didn't do as well after the second session as she had on the first. Her pain level when she came in was 7 on the 0-10 pain scale. As I began my ZB evaluation and treatment, I again experienced many areas of tension and sluggishness throughout TC's body. I performed a 40-minute ZB protocol. I did extra work on her hips and added special neck fulcrums. I suggested that she continue with ZB sessions since she had seen some positive changes with this modality.

TC's fourth visit took place three and a half months after her third ZB session. She reported now using arnica cream on her legs on a daily basis. Since the last treatment, she reported that she was able to sleep through the night. The predominate tension pattern I felt on this visit was at T-4-5-6 in her thoracic cage. As usual, her tibias and fibulas were dense, her Achilles tendons were dense and tight, and her neck glide was sluggish. I performed a 30-minute ZB on her. I added additional fulcrums to her tibias, fibulas and ankles. I continued to use special neck fulcrums. The tension in her thoracic cage eased by approximately 50%. Her neck glide opened by about 10%. The client stated that she felt great after the session.

TC came for her fifth visit the following month. She said she was still doing well and considered herself to be here for maintenance ZB. She said she continued to feel great with ZB. "I am amazed, after seeing so many physicians...that ZB is the only thing that has helped my legs."

In general, I have seen TC once a month for the past two years. I still focus on her tibias, fibulas and Achilles tendons since they continue to hold tension.

When TC has not been able to do monthly ZB sessions she has experienced increased leg pain. She feels that as long as she can receive ZB once a month, her leg pain is either gone or not as noticeable or bothersome–and that she can sleep through the night!

Practitioner: Maureen Staudt, BSN, RN, LMT, CZB
Modalities: Zero Balancing
ZB Experience: Studying ZB since 2004, certified in 2006, ZB mentor, ZB faculty
Location: Souderton, PA

• • •

"She said ZB has been the only treatment to date that has given her relief from the pain."

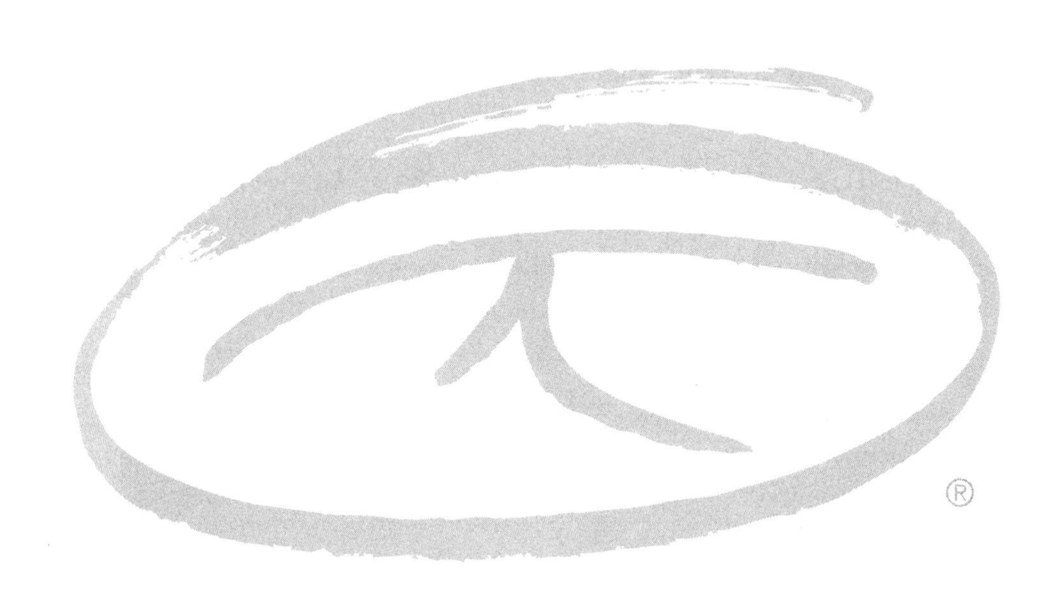

Working with the Emotion of Anger

Maureen Staudt, BSN, RN, LMT, CZB

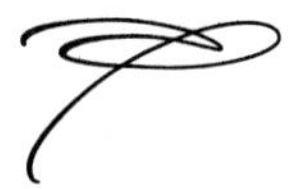

BACKGROUND

Bill was 26 years old when he came for his first Zero Balancing treatment. His mother, who is a client of mine, referred him to me, and his older brother accompanied him to this appointment. Bill and his brother work at a factory where they cut and carve soapstone.

ZERO BALANCING

When I asked Bill how he wanted to feel after the session was over, he said, "I want to feel less angry." I wanted to make the session comfortable and non-threatening for both Bill and his brother. I therefore decided not to ask any questions regarding this anger that Bill was feeling. As for me, the practitioner, the first thought that came to me was, "Gee, what am I going to do about anger?" As quickly as I questioned myself I remembered to trust the ZB protocol.

On evaluation, the quality of Bill's voice suggested low energy and I noticed that his eyes were twitching. The knuckles in both his hands were dense and heavy; those on his left hand were reddened and his thoracic area was very heavy and dense, but his neck range of motion was full and free. (I assumed these physical findings were most likely due to the work he does at the factory.)

I performed a 40-minute session on Bill. I suggested that he be kind to himself, to notice any small changes during the next 24 to 48 hours, and to call me with any concerns or questions.

A week later, Bill came for his second visit. He stated that he felt improvement since his first ZB. He said his anger was not as noticeable and that little things that usually annoyed him did not bother him as much. He told me that his boss told him that whatever he changed this past week, he should, "keep it up." His mother also asked what I had done to him because she noticed he was significantly less angry since receiving his first ZB.

I continued to see Bill weekly for the next three months. Although he reported some ups and downs regarding feelings of stress and irritation, he repeatedly reported noticing that he did not get angry as easily as he did before ZB. His frame for each session was essentially the same: "I want to feel the same as I did after the last ZB; to feel stress-free." I also taught him a "marching in place" technique that we use in ZB that helps one feel more grounded after a session. Bill found this to be helpful and practiced this technique at the end of each session.

Due to the strenuous, physical nature of his job, Bill continued to have tension in his shoulders and scapula. During these sessions he admitted to me that he had lost jobs in the past due to his anger issues. He said his current boss at the soapstone factory was so impressed by the change in him that he wanted me to come to the company and work on everyone. Bill also commented that his co-workers had also noticed an improvement in his anger and "crabbiness."

I continued to work with Bill, as needed, throughout the next three years. Each time he came in he would say something like, "I am glad I am here today. I know that ZB will help me." And it always did.

I will say that when he first came to me and asked to feel less angry, I really stepped back and wondered how I could help him. By trusting the ZB protocol I allowed myself to get out of the way. Bill showed me that one cannot only bring physical goals to a session but one can bring emotional or spiritual goals as well.

Practitioner: Maureen Staudt, BSN, RN, LMT, CZB

Modalities: Zero Balancing

ZB Experience: Studying ZB since 2004, certified in 2006, ZB mentor, ZB faculty

Location: Souderton, PA

• • •

"During these sessions he admitted to me that he had lost jobs in the past due to his anger issues."

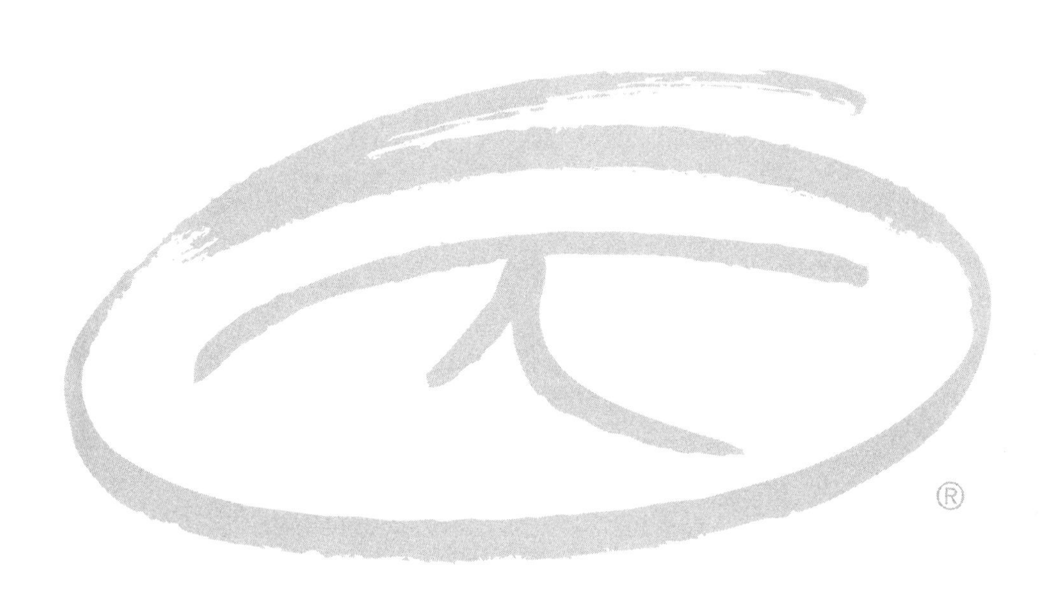

Chronic Pain from Old Injuries: A Client's Testimony

Judith Sullivan, BS, BCTMB, CST, CZB

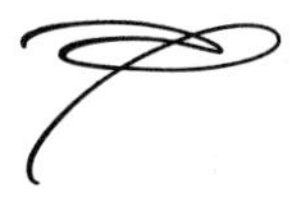

BACKGROUND

I am 45 years old, and have had chronic neck, jaw, shoulder, and thoracic rib pain for many years. Having never been in a major accident, I had decided that I must suffer from a genetic predisposition that causes me to go out of alignment on a regular basis. I felt that I was stuck like this for life. The idea of feeling pain for the rest of my life was very emotionally and psychologically debilitating, which only compounded the actual physical discomfort. I have two small children, and was not able to be as active or in shape as I would like.

ZERO BALANCING

I started working with Judith Sullivan about eight months ago, and after receiving regular Zero Balancing, I currently feel more "normal" in my body than I have in years. I have also been doing regular Pilates, and seeing an osteopath for about four years, but the work with Judith has taken me over the finish line. I recall asking her if she could help me with my ribs, as I did not think that rib work was typical. She laughed and replied, "Some people have called me the Rib Maven." That is when I knew I was in the right place! The journey with Judith has been very interesting.

I recalled several seemingly insignificant accidents that seemed to have done some long-term damage to my body. The earliest of these accidents happened when I was twelve years old. I was on the tennis court and blacked out from heat stroke. My braces catching on the chain link fence broke my fall. When I woke up, my mouth was cut up, and while the braces were still on my teeth, the bands were ripped open and sticking out of my mouth. The most amazing thing was when Judith started working on my teeth, all of this came back to me. This fall had clearly done some damage to my neck and jaw, possibly even caused some hairline fractures in the bones of my mouth. By releasing some of that blocked energy from those teeth, my neck and jaw pain is gone!

The next injury I experienced was when I fell off a rope swing while rafting down the Chattahoochee River and landed on the shore, only to bounce another 15 feet on my bottom into the water. It was funny at the time, but I probably fractured my coccyx bone during the fall. Working on my coccyx bone and lower sacral vertebrae has allowed my body to be in better alignment, which helps in every way!

The final accident is the one that probably caused my most painful problem–the pain of my ribs moving out of position all of the time. When I was in college, I offered a male friend a piggyback ride back to the dorms from a frat party. You get the picture. He got a running start and jumped on my back. My knees buckled, and I fell to the sidewalk. I broke my left arm, and now realize that I might have fractured some ribs as well. Judith and I are still working on my ribs, but my pain has gone from a roar to a whisper, which is the most wonderful and liberating outcome I could ever hope for!

Needless to say, my whole family has seen Judith for various ailments and accidents. I do not want my children to feel pain later in life from something we missed while they were children! – K.F.

Practitioner: Judith Sullivan, BS in Education, Speech Pathology and Audiology, graduate work in Psychology, BCTMB, CST (Certified CranioSacral Therapy Diplomate Therapist by the Upledger Institute), CZB

Modalities: Zero Balancing and CranioSacral Therapy

ZB Experience: Studying ZB since 1983, certified in 1989, ZB faculty, Director of Certification (2002-2008), editor of the Core Zero Balancing Study Guide with Dr. Fritz Smith, Vice President of the ZBHA Board of Directors until 2014

Location: Charlottesville, VA

Forty Years of Migraines from Hell: A Client's Testimony

Judith Sullivan, BS, BCTMB, CST, CZB

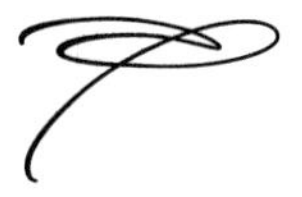

BACKGROUND

CB first came to see me when she was about 60 years old. Describing herself as a "housewife," CB had been suffering from "migraines from hell," as well as chronic fatigue and fibromyalgia for over forty years. Because her energy was so low, her husband drove her from their home to my office in Charlottesville, Virginia a four-hour trip. I saw her for about a year, during which time her headaches steadily improved and finally "broke." CB then continued to see me approximately once every three months for maintenance over a period of two more years. Later on, I referred her to a ZB practitioner in her own city.

CB'S STORY:

When I started receiving Zero Balancing, I wasn't convinced that another new treatment would really help my migraine headaches. Having had migraines for forty years and finding no lasting relief from previous medications, hospitalizations, and therapy, I was open to try ZB.

The first few times Judith worked with me, there was a change in my headaches, and in general I experienced improvement. However, a few times the treatments made the pain worse. Judith's encouragement and statement that if she could "make my headaches worse, she could make them better," convinced me to give ZB a fair trial. I made a commitment to make a four-hour drive every two weeks to Charlottesville and also to do a three-day visit to Charlottesville for two intensive sessions a day.

I began to have fewer severe headaches and was able to decrease and then discontinue several medications I had been on for many years.

At this point, I have very few headaches and the intensity has decreased tremendously. I am excited and pleased with the progress we have made. I am very grateful that Judith has helped me regain my health. I am truly thankful for her knowledge of ZB and I am especially grateful for her healing hands. – CB

Practitioner: Judith Sullivan, BS in Education, Speech Pathology and Audiology, graduate work in Psychology, BCTMB, CST (Certified CranioSacral Therapy Diplomate Therapist by the Upledger Institute), CZB

Modalities: Zero Balancing and CranioSacral Therapy

ZB Experience: Studying ZB since 1983, certified in 1989, ZB faculty, Director of Certification (2002-2008), editor of the Core Zero Balancing Study Guide with Dr. Fritz Smith, Vice President of the ZBHA Board of Directors until 2014

Location: Charlottesville, VA

• • •

"When there is an issue in the body, somewhere there is another end of the string." — Fritz Frederick Smith, MD

Zero Balancing Deepens the Spiritual Direction Experience

Deanna Waggy, OTR, CZB

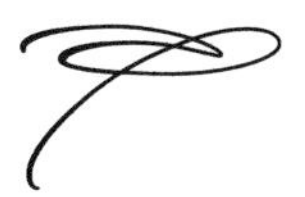

There are many ways to accompany others on their spiritual journey, such as pastoral counseling, spiritual direction, healing guidance and shamanic healing. Most of these forms of accompaniment involve meeting "one with one" or in small group discussions. This work involves exploring unresolved issues of the heart and inner landscapes.

After receiving Zero Balancing training, I began offering my clients a combination of ZB and spiritual direction. Some clients noticed a difference with the depth of their inner work when they had a ZB session first, followed by a spiritual direction session. They noticed that ZB was able to help them reach expanded states of consciousness and address the inner issues at a deeper level.

Naturally curious, I decided to focus on my own issues related to my inner heart during the next ZB session I received. I set a frame (intention) for the session related to opening up my heart to be more loving and accepting of others. While the ZB practitioner was working on my shoulder blades, I experienced growing warmth in my chest, followed by a bright white light filling my whole chest cavity. It was difficult to breathe as if someone was tightly squeezing my chest. When I verbalized this, the ZB practitioner lifted me up off the table under my shoulder blades and encouraged me to "let go of all that no longer serves you." As I exhaled, she slowly lowered me to the table and I felt lightness as if my heart were floating on water followed by a deep sense of joy bubbling up from deep within me. I met later with my spiritual director for further exploration and insight. These feelings of lightheartedness, overwhelming tenderness and joy lasted for several weeks.

Several friends wanted to experience this combination of ZB and spiritual direction. Three of the four women had significant experiences.

One woman focused on her Enneagram type during her ZB session. She then followed up with her spiritual director the next day. She reported new insights from that session, even though she had been attending various workshops and working with her director for many years. She continues to come for ZB sessions prior to her spiritual direction sessions whenever she feels she is ready to move deeper during her inner work.

One woman wanted to, "release any past hurts that are hindering me." I did the Core ZB protocol with her. Near the end of her session I intuitively added fulcrums to her sternum to open her heart to awareness of past hurts. While placing fulcrums into the sternum, she began to sob. She began praying in Polish, then eventually breathed a deep sigh and smiled. After the ZB session she said that she had a growing awareness of the deep grief and pain her ancestors suffered in concentration camps during WWII. She also realized her need to forgive those who had tortured and killed her ancestors, thus her prayers in her native tongue. She has had subsequent ZB sessions, but none as profound as this first experience.

Another woman had been working with her spiritual director through her 50-year-old unresolved grief from two untimely deaths of a boyfriend and older brother when she was a teenager. She told me she felt as if she were taking baby steps in her grief work. She set a frame for her ZB session so that she could, "open up and dig deeper into this old grief that has been pushed down inside of me all these years." I used the standard ZB protocol for her session. She had some signs that she was going into a deep expanded state of awareness, including muscle twitches, rapid eye movements and occasional deep breaths. She also had a single tear roll down her cheek near the end of the session. After her ZB session, she confessed that she had been unable to cry for these young men after their deaths. Near the end of the session, she had the sense they were both present in the room with us, which was a sign of encouragement for her to keep unearthing her feelings and grief. She was also encouraged by the fact that tears were welling up within her for the first time since these losses. She was able to follow up with her spiritual director for further inner work within a few days and expressed gratitude that she had, "unearthed some layers because of the ZB session."

While facilitating a one-day retreat last year on the topic of self-care, I offered short 15-minute ZB sessions to several regular retreat participants during their morning silent reflection time. The participants felt the ZB helped them relax deeper into their meditation time. Their openness and depth of vulnerability during the group session later that afternoon confirmed a deeper level of spiritual awareness, compared to the other retreat days they attended during this monthly retreat series. Since this time, I try to provide short ZB sessions as an option either before or during the spiritual retreats I facilitate. When I do not offer ZB sessions with the retreats, the women often ask if I can give them a short session anyway, as they miss having it as part of the retreat experience.

From these experiences, I have observed that the combination of a ZB session followed by a spiritual direction session has helped many people to experience a deeper level of spiritual growth than one of these sessions alone. This was also observed with short ZB sessions during a spiritual retreat. I will continue to offer this combination to those interested in inner work and spiritual growth.

Author's note: *Spiritual Direction has been around for thousands of years, and goes by many names depending on which spiritual tradition you come from. Spiritual Directors International is a global community for those who provide spiritual companionship services. It is hard to define Spiritual Direction because there are so many diverse traditions that use this model of one-to-one companionship, and it can take many forms depending on the needs of the individual. For more information, see http://www.sdiworld.org/find-a-spiritual-director/what-is-spiritual-direction*

Spiritual Direction (sometimes called mentoring, guidance or coaching) explores a deeper relationship with the spiritual aspect of being human. Simply put, Spiritual

Direction is helping people tell their sacred stories. It is not talk therapy. It is not counseling. It is not about our horizontal relationships with others. It is about our vertical relationship with the Divine. As people begin the process of spiritual awakening, they may want a companion on their spiritual journey. Spiritual Direction is sometimes referred to as, "tending the holy," or a, "midwife for the soul." These mentors typically meet one-to-one with people as they awake to the mystery of the Divine in their life.

Practitioner: Deanna Waggy, OTR, CZB
Modalities: Occupational Therapy and Zero Balancing
ZB experiences: Studying ZB since 2011, certified in 2011, ZB mentor
Location: South Bend, IN

• • •

"One woman wanted to, 'release any past hurts that are hindering me.' "

Zero Balancing with Asperger Syndrome/ Autism Spectrum

Deanna Waggy, OTR, CZB

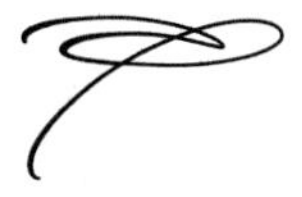

BACKGROUND

Sonia is a 24-year-old diagnosed with Sensory Processing Disorder, Autism and Asperger Syndrome. She lives with her parents and attends college part-time. She must maintain a minimum of twelve credits in order to keep her scholarships, which is a constant struggle for her. She is taking a ballet class for credit to help relieve the academic load, provide exercise and foster body awareness, even though she struggles with balance and coordination. Sonia suffers from chronic migraines, which have been getting progressively worse despite seeing various specialists. She is overweight, depressed and overwhelmed with basic daily living skills. She also has poor social skills, difficulty concentrating, poor sleep habits and emotional outbursts.

ZERO BALANCING

Sonia's goal for her first few Zero Balancing sessions was to decrease the intensity and frequency of her migraines. Each time, I used the Core ZB protocol, noticing areas of dense energy and tension in her pelvic region, feet, shoulders and neck. Sonia held her body in a rigid, guarded posture throughout the first few sessions. When I picked up her feet for the initial Half Moon Vector (HMV), she locked her hips and knees and resisted movement. I remained grounded to hold a clear strong field until I felt changes in her held tension for each fulcrum (gentle finger pressure held for a few seconds to create a balance point around which the body can reorient). By the end of each session she was relaxed and allowed the fulcrums without tensing up.

As her migraines diminished, Sonia added additional goals for the sessions, including improved balance in ballet class and better concentration in her other classes. I added fulcrums to the jaw area to release tension from clenched teeth, rib fulcrums to address the shallow breathing, neck fulcrums to increase neck motion and skull fulcrums to help with whole brain learning, right/left integration and concentration. I also added additional foot fulcrums to improve her grounding and balance for ballet and shoulder girdle fulcrums to improve her coordination and ability to function in the world.

After the first several sessions, Sonia noticed the following improvements: decreased frequency and intensity of her migraines, improved spatial awareness during jumps in ballet, improved concentration for studies and the ability to relax more quickly. Sonia's mother reported amazing improvement in Sonia's grades from C's to A's in all her classes. I noticed improved, less guarded posture, a greater ease of movement, an increased lung capacity, a quicker relaxation response, improved social interactions, direct eye contact, and parasympathetic nervous system responses (working signs) during sessions.

Her mother wrote to me:

> *Sonia is very worried about carrying twelve credits this semester. She sees all of her family and friends moving on and doing things, and is so very sensitive to being left behind. I've known her to be upset, but never anxious or worried about the future. Autistic kids are known for living only in the moment. This whole framework of being aware of time outside of the present is a very new phenomenon. I think it is a good thing, but it is like watching her awaken from a dream only to find that the whole world has moved on while she slept. For so many years, she's been lost–submerged in a dark environment without distinctive features, with no predictability and all out of her control. Since working with you, I see her discerning ways and places to make choices, and that her choices have the power to change reality. Instead of always burrowing down in*

the murky depths to find security and safety, she has found that there are other choices that can be made to actually change things for the better.

Sonia took a six-week break from ZB over the winter holidays. During this break she experienced a noticeable regression in her symptoms and several "spectacular meltdowns," according to her mother. She requested more ZB sessions.

On the next visit I discovered extremely dense energy throughout the pelvis, feet and neck. Her energy felt like a tightly wound spring throughout her body and she moved in robotic-like movements. Her goal was to "make it through the rest of the week at school." She was nervous about keeping up with classes due to the return of her migraines. She wanted to experience the good feeling through ZB that she had experienced the previous semester. I began again with the basic ZB protocol with a few integrating fulcrums to the skull. I placed extra focus on being grounded to give her a sense of stability.

After this session, her mother wrote:

> *Look what your ZB has done: Sonia was so relaxed and happy when she left her ZB session. She finally slept well, and the five-day long headache broke overnight. Earlier this week, she could not bathe herself, fix a meal, or concentrate on reading a simple young adult novel. Her verbal responses were two words. She slept a lot, was very fragile and irritable and discouraged. Needless to say, she could not study or take coherent notes in class during this time. This morning, she woke up without a headache. She had lots of good eye contact and a begrudging willingness to buckle down for a time to try to get a couple of philosophy assignments together. She wrote her assignment in about ten minutes using complex sentences and higher level thought processes.*

Sonia wants to continue with ZB on a regular basis. I am interested in empowering Sonia to learn additional self-care strategies such as Yin

Yoga, Tai Chi or Qigong between ZB sessions so she does not become dependent on ZB. From a conventional medicine perspective, Sonia has a complex history and a myriad of problems, which interfere with her ability to function on a daily basis. Through ZB, we are beginning to see a cocoon splitting open and a butterfly slowly starting to emerge. Sonia's response suggests that ZB gives new possibilities for people living on the autism spectrum.

Practitioner: Deanna Waggy, OTR, CZB
Modalities: Occupational Therapy and Zero Balancing
ZB experiences: Studying ZB since 2011, certified in 2011, ZB mentor
Location: South Bend, IN

• • •

"As her migraines diminished, Sonia added additional goals for the sessions, including improved balance and better concentration."

It's OK to be Me?!!!

Cassie White, PA, MT, CZB

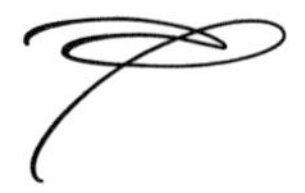

BACKGROUND

AB came to me for Zero Balancing to let go of the past and to find more balance in her life, wanting to be more of herself, whatever that was! A young woman in her late thirties, she was working hard juggling a part-time job around caring for her healthy and very energetic four-year-old son, together with coming to terms with a recent divorce. Her ex-husband was a registered gambler and alcoholic. Having met her soul mate after this event and with the complexities that extended families can experience, AB was feeling overwhelmed and out of sorts. This manifested in her feeling "low." Physically, she was "bearing up" and still managing her exercise and time at the gym, although it wasn't as much fun. Headaches were becoming more of an everyday thing. AB's work involved coaching others with obesity and eating disorders. She has had years of counseling and psychotherapy herself and was looking to integrate the work she had already done so she could become happy being herself.

ZERO BALANCING

AB's voice was very soft spoken and would often trail off, as did her stare whilst talking. She walked silently and often on tip toe and, when asked if there was any significant event that had happened other than her divorce, a blank stare and shake of the head was the response.

I explained that ZB was worked through clothing, was non-invasive and non-diagnostic. I let her know that I was not there to mend, fix or change anything. Her soul and body wisdom had all she needed to bring her back into balance and in harmony with her choices.

Her first session was 20 minutes, whereby I followed the basic ZB protocol. There was no frame or intention as AB had shared in detail her current situation and it was enough to simply have a ZB.

As I began, I was aware that her energy body felt fractured and, whilst her energy moved quickly and freely, it was without a container. As I evaluated her lower body I felt there was an area of held energy in her pelvic region and in her lower spine. AB's skin colour changed as I worked, turning from waxen and pale to having a soft glow just like a gorgeous new rosy apple in its first flush. Throughout the session, soft half smiles would appear on her face. With each one I paused to allow her to silently have the experience for herself. As I worked the top half of her body she seemed to literally come alive on my fingertips. When I asked how she was doing, a clear and much stronger voice announced, "Fine! It's all about boundaries!" As the session came to a close, this young woman looked very different from the one who had arrived. As she walked up and down the room after the session she beamed with her whole body. "This is what I have been looking for and my own answers just came to me!"

AB received ZB sessions once a month for eight months with a gap of two months, after which she received monthly sessions again. Each session would last about an hour with a chat before each one. The ZB was usually 20 to 40 minutes long with a moment after the session to empower the changes that came into her awareness.

The second session saw her stride into my room with far more confidence and with a clearer understanding of what she really wanted, even if she had no clue as to how to get there! Relationships were starting to become more structured with routines and boundaries in place, and her voice was clear and instructive. She loved her job but wanted to feel heard and valued by her colleagues. AB wanted to have some stability with her son's visits with his father, and she wanted to be more open in her new relationship, letting go of fear and building on what she felt in her heart and soul, and not what she thought she ought to do based on old perceptions. Her headaches were gone but a lower backache had shown itself. “I have stayed more grounded since I last saw you, which is so good to feel and makes my life easier.”

Her frame was to move forward easily and to have things improve. Which they did. By her fifth session an abusive and cruel incident as a teenager revealed itself and, during her session, AB was able to feel and see its total release. Her body relaxed and softened as I worked with her energy body becoming whole and having the quality of liquid gold.

The next three sessions enabled her to come to terms with how new she felt and how much more in control of her own life she was. It has been a gift to watch this woman learn to speak up, remain grounded, own her likes and dislikes and just witness them. Her backache cleared totally. She had gone through menopause in seven months and was now on HRT. Tiredness ensued, leaving her unable to exercise and with her doctor flagging up all the ailments of post-menopause.

AB came to me after a two-month gap as she felt unheard and negated. I gently let her know that after such a big transformation the body sometimes needs rest. With this she laughed and said, “I have been driving it hard for a long time!” AB had just been offered the job of her dreams and was aware that this had come to her once she really understood that she had to listen to herself and not override what she knew! Her relationship with her little boy was better than ever and everything was moving forward in the right direction. Her frame was to let her body know she was now listening to herself and acting on it. Once again I followed the basic ZB protocol, and as the session continued this woman became more beautiful and relaxed. When I asked her halfway through the session how she was her reply was, “Fabulous!”

I asked her to repeat that so all her body could hear her. “I AM fabulous!” she said as it rang around the room with the resonance of a singing bowl. I closed the session, and as she sat up she said, “I am Present.” I invited her to walk her presence into the moment she was in being fabulous. She walked easily, grounded and relaxed, and, as she did so, smiled and said, "I am aligned, truly aligned and I am home. Thank you. ZB has allowed me to transform myself. It's OK to be me!"

Practitioner: Cassie White, ITEC, MT, Adv PA, CZB
Modalities: Massage Therapy, Process Acupressure, Zero Balancing
ZB experience: Studying ZB since 1997, certified in 1999, ZB faculty
Location: Ferring, West Sussex, UK

• • •

"It has been a gift to watch this woman learn to speak up, remain grounded, own her likes and dislikes and just witness them."

Embodiment

Todd Williams, CMT, CZB

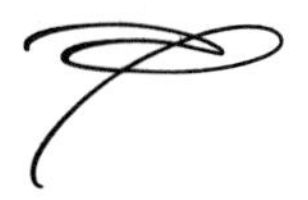

BACKGROUND

Simon is a 60-year-old male. He came to ZB in an unusual way. He told me that he opened his date book one day and found "Zero Balancing" written down. He had no recollection of anyone telling him about it or when or where he may have heard about it. He looked it up on the Internet, found my listing and contacted me. His reason for coming was that he wanted to be more "embodied." He presented with no physical complaints, but was open to exploring bodywork as a way to know himself more deeply and fully in his body. Simon had previously received Rolfing and massage work, as well as psychotherapy. He also follows a spiritual path and has a meditation practice.

ZERO BALANCING

Simon received a total of 19 ZB sessions.

First session

From the outset this was a fascinating session. At the very beginning it seemed to be a sheer joy for Simon to feel touched at the core level of bone tissue. He verbally expressed his happiness at being touched in the ZB way. During the session I would find a spot of held tension in bone, or excess vibration as we say in ZB, and hold it for a few seconds creating a fulcrum (a stable point around which the body can reorient). I also touched him in such a way that would feel as good as possible to him. In those moments Simon would make a deep "ah" sound and sometimes say, "it feels so good." Often as I would hold a point, there would be a response in his body such as a shake or quiver. Some of these body movements I would describe as Kriyas. (The word Kriya means "action" in Sanskrit and comes from the Hindu Yoga philosophy. It can be used to denote the movement of Shakti or vibration through one or many of the 72,000 nadis, or channels of life force in the human body. In ZB terms a Kriya is considered to be a working sign by which we read the body's response to the touch and monitor the integration of energy with body structure, particularly bone tissue). By the end of the first session when Simon lay on the table, he said, "It feels like coming home to myself. Where have I been all this time?!" There were tears of joy.

Patterns and shifts

Working with Simon over the next month I noticed a distinct pattern of held tension in his left upper ribcage and shoulder girdle. It felt as though he were guarding himself against something. I also found that the ribs and shoulder girdle related directly to the alignment of the pelvic bones and the energy flow through the lower body. Many fulcrums would allow body movements to occur in his pelvis and legs, which appeared to be a re-organization or re-patterning.

Each session represented a profound body-mind shift for Simon. There were comments such as, "Feels like an electrical current has been switched on. I didn't know my body could feel like this–awake and electric." At one point Simon said he began to "see" the energy inside his body in the sides of his pelvis and hip joints when he sat for his meditations. He reported a process he went through after sessions at home, laying on his bed quietly letting his body "quake." He said it felt good and also described feeling more vitality in his body, "like a teenager." He also said he was aware of his entire skeleton and that he could feel how much it supported him and felt strong. He began exercising regularly and enjoyed physical movement to a greater degree. Each session seemed to take him on an upward curve toward greater health and vitality.

Imagery, body sensations and armoring

As we continued to work, Simon said he was aware of his having a layer of protection in his body that didn't need to be there. He also reported feeling freer and easier around people at work, yet noticed the times when his body armoring was "back on." At this point in our work, Simon became slightly depressed, reporting moodiness and having been "in a fog," feeling not himself and stuck. He said his body felt heavy, especially his lower body. He reported that his left shoulder had felt stiff and sore and he could not and did not want to exercise. Work on the left rib cage and shoulder girdle continued to be significant. As I placed fulcrums here, Simon reported an image of a steel rod, like a support in a cement structure, inside his left chest and arm. This appeared for several sessions. As we continued to work on this area the image of molten lava would appear. He experienced a release of heat from his entire body. Working signs included increased heart rate and profuse sweating which was not typical. There was some disorientation during the session and afterward in walking but gradually he felt stable.

Release of old patterns and toxins

In one particular session there was a smell of smoke from the street below, which came in through the open window just before we began our work. It was unusual, and Simon and I both remarked on it. I didn't know what the significance was at the time, but I have learned to pay attention to synchronistic events in my field of awareness such as sounds, smells, environmental changes in light or temperature. They may be related to something the client is experiencing. During this session it became clear that breath was a key to making the next step toward embodiment. As I touched his ribs, held fulcrums and moved from point to point, Simon would take deep breaths. He commented that he was aware of "breathing in life," and how closely linked to vitality is the breath. At one point in this session as I held a fulcrum, Simon said he had a metallic taste in his mouth. This dissipated and returned a second time in the session. Later a smell of smoke was discernible to me. It seemed like a releasing, cleansing process occurred during the session as the costo-vertebral joints became freer and more balanced, and lung capacity increased. After the session Simon commented that he had been a smoker for many years, but it had been twenty or more years since he'd quit.

Integration

Simon came to the session describing events after our previous session. He said the session had "stayed with him" for several days. He went to a restaurant after the session for a favorite meal. The next day he got food poisoning as a result of some undercooked fish. He described being able to fully accept the process of being sick temporarily as he witnessed the wisdom in the body "knowing what to do." When it was over he felt good and was able to appreciate being both perfectly healthy and temporarily ill as part of the whole. He was eager, curious and excited to see how his next session would unfold.

During the first part of this ZB I asked Simon how he was feeling. He said he wanted to be fully present but was noticing his mind going back and forth from thoughts to body sensations. I asked him to bring all of his attention to my fingers making contact with his body (at the left sacroiliac joint). This brought his attention to how each touch felt during the session. One significant fulcrum here yielded a Kriya, which he described as "like lightning moving through me." As I worked on his lower limbs he remarked that he was aware of "how important they are and how much work they do to hold me up." At another point I asked him what he was experiencing and he said, "I'm aware that I'm looking for the part of me that is 'not good.' I'm hoping you can find it."

I continued the session. When I reached the upper body portion of the session he said he felt his armoring again, "like a football player with shoulder pads." As I touched his upper trapezius, scapulae and clavicles, there was a palpable dense vibration in them. The instant feedback was, "Oh, that's it . . . it's so tense." As I put fulcrums into the shoulder girdle he described his internal imagery about his armoring changing into a "Samurai." He said, "I like this energy and it feels so good!" I encouraged him verbally to feel it in his entire body. While I held one fulcrum on the trapezius and shoulder girdle longer than usual, Simon moved his legs like he was walking, letting them flop down with all their weight onto the table. As the session went on he described the colors red and black along with a feeling of robust power. He said, "I feel there's no room for any bad belief system about myself–get out!" When he got off the table, he strode purposefully and confidently, appearing grounded and aligned. He said, "I feel completely present and in my body. It feels like a good place to be."

Sessions will continue with Simon, as he is excited to learn more about embodiment and how the ZB work can further assist him.

Practitioner: Todd Williams, CMT, CZB

Modalities: Certified Massage Therapist, Zero Balancing

ZB experience: Studying ZB since 1999, certified in 2007, ZB mentor, ZB faculty, ZBHA Board of Directors Co-Chair

Location: San Francisco Bay Area, CA

• • •

"Simon reported an image of a steel rod, like a support in a cement structure, inside his left chest and arm."

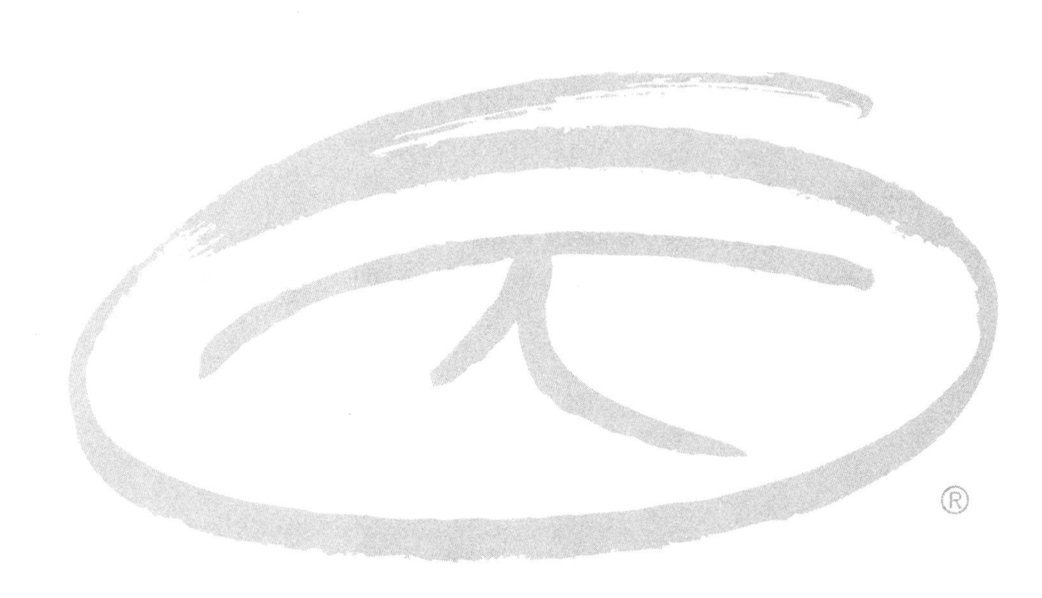

Psychotherapy and Zero Balancing: A Potent Synergy

Anne Wissler, LCSW, CMT, CYT, CZB

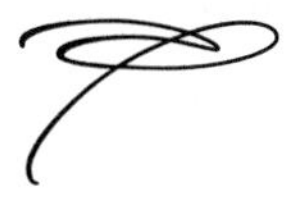

BACKGROUND

My first impressions of Zero Balancing, first as a receiver, and then as practitioner, sparked a vision of its potential to catalyze inner growth by accessing a felt sense of one's fundamental wholeness. Often, people with trauma histories are so organized to protect and defend that their very identity is woven into patterns of limitation. The defensive matrix, contrived to outside awareness to keep them safe, can deny direct access to their own wholeness and peace. By contacting primal bone-held energy, ZB reaches safely below the cognitive personality matrix, inviting an experience of one's original nature that is not entangled within this limiting matrix. This deep knowing helps to hold the caught or limited self in a bigger energy field as it softens, releases and reorganizes, freeing the receiver to continue to evolve.

From this vision, one client stood out as a good candidate for receiving ZB in conjunction with her psychotherapy growth process. At the time, MJ was a 45-year-old married artist and writer. She had a history of trauma, anxiety, and fatigue with debilitating body tensions, panic attacks, disrupted sleep patterns, food allergies, and racing thoughts. Incapacitating fear-based clenching patterns often hijacked her body, generating pain, draining her energy, and escalating physical and emotional sensitivity. Her strong capacity for self-reflection served to develop a good understanding of various limiting patterns. And yet listening to her, I could not detect her sense of being at home in her body, that reservoir of wholeness that I knew was there. But did she?

While new to practicing ZB, I offered it from my persisting sense that it could allow MJ access to that substrate of well-being sealed off by an over-active intellect. Introducing ZB to her, I said that it balances energy with structure, organizing, clarifying and freeing bone-held energy to be recycled back into her system, and that often people find ZB deeply meditative and relaxing. Given that these ideas were familiar to her from yoga, she was eager to explore this modality.

ZERO BALANCING

We began with three sessions one week apart to acquaint her with the work and begin to build on its effects. We minimized talking and kept a simple frame for each session: to explore the experience of receiving ZB. Initially, she was pleased and curious at how relaxed she could feel. Given the working relationship of trust we already had, she was energetically open and receptive to the work, even though her intellect could neither direct nor account for its effects. Instead, she was challenged to rely more on her embodied experience, a less familiar channel of knowing.

From these three sessions, she decided to continue to receive ZB on an average of once every three weeks. Suspending expectations for immediate results, our overriding intention was to build a reservoir of experience of the inherent stability underlying the taxing, trauma-based ways she protects herself. Still, useful effects were immediate: a solidness experienced in the legs, which persistently conveyed sensations of groundedness, purveying a confidence that showed up in her posture; physical/bodily sensations supported a moment-by-moment choice to explore, rather than block feelings, thus reducing internal pressure of feelings building up. Correspondingly, I noticed a positive back-and-forth loosening or re-shuffling through her energy field while giving the ZB. These changes appeared to have a profound effect on our psychotherapy sessions—MJ was now softening into feeling instead of intellectually distancing herself.

At six months, I was surprised and touched by the spontaneous emerging of soundings from her depths. She stopped the self-imposed "workouts" she'd hated, replacing them with forms of exercise that nourished her. She tolerated the "fuzzy-headedness" that sometimes occurs when making deep energetic shifts in ZB. This led to tolerance of the inevitable uncertainty and chaos within the creative cycle of her work. Her frames for the sessions became clearer and more succinct, rather than convoluted. During one ZB session, it dawned on her that she'd been sleeping more soundly, having turned off the white noise machine she had needed to manage noise sensitivity, forgetting about it for some months. From this most basic shift into a deeper knowing of herself, MJ was freeing herself to continue to evolve and allow the flow of nervous system recovery to take place. This could then have a positive, beneficial effect on cognitive function, relational resilience and rolling with life's uncertainties. Less worried by how and when her body might "crash" and pull her back from life, her physical stress signals became more localized, and MJ had a means for self-understanding and compassion through the inner work of psychotherapy.

As she settled into understanding her body, rather than fearing it, the psychotherapy process naturally accelerated. She brought more resilience and self-trust to proactively working within the relational sphere. She began to schedule ZB sessions when she wanted access to her creative inspirations, or to get unstuck in her process. While there is no way to say what might have occurred in the same year without ZB, I was surprised when MJ took a leap "ahead of schedule" as compared to non-ZB clients. A threshold was crossed and stabilized from which she demonstrated a gratifying, deep-rooted trust in herself.

From this experience, I can see other situations in which ZB is likely to be a catalyst for growth and change, by giving people more access to themselves at a deep level. Additionally, I have no doubt that clients of mine, who have not directly experienced ZB, have still benefited indirectly from the deep peace and joy that ZB has brought to me over the year as a receiver. To go beneath the cognitive personality level and bask in the wellsprings of wisdom grants the conviction of unity and integrity that colors all of human life more richly and expansively, while grounding in its simplicity.

Practitioner: Anne Wissler, LCSW, CMT, Cert. Yoga Therapy, CZB

Modalities: Zero Balancing, Integrative Psychotherapist and Couples Therapy since 1976, Yoga Instructor since 1996

ZB experience: Studying ZB since 2012, certified in 2014

Location: Atlanta, GA

• • •

"These changes appeared to have a profound effect on our psychotherapy sessions—MJ was now softening into feeling instead of intellectually distancing herself."

References

Hamwee, John, *Zero Balancing: Touching the Energy of Bone*, Singing Dragon, 2014

Smith, Fritz Frederick, MD, *Inner Bridges: A Guide to Energy Movement and Body Structure*, Humanics Limited, 1986

Smith, Fritz Frederick, MD, *The Alchemy of Touch: Moving Towards Mastery through the Lens of Zero Balancing*, Complementary Medicine Press, 2005

Sullivan, Judith, *Zero Balancing Expanded: The Attitude of Awaiting a Fish*, Upledger Productions, 2014

For more information about Zero Balancing, or to contact these or other certified Zero Balancing practitioners, please visit the following websites:

North America:
www.zerobalancing.com
www.iahp.com

United Kingdom
www.zerobalancinguk.com

Italy
www.zerobalancing.it

Mexico
www.balanceceromexico.com

New Zealand/Australia
www.zerobalancing.co.nz

Switzerland
www.zerobalancing.ch

Zero Balancing Touch Foundation
www.zbtouch.org

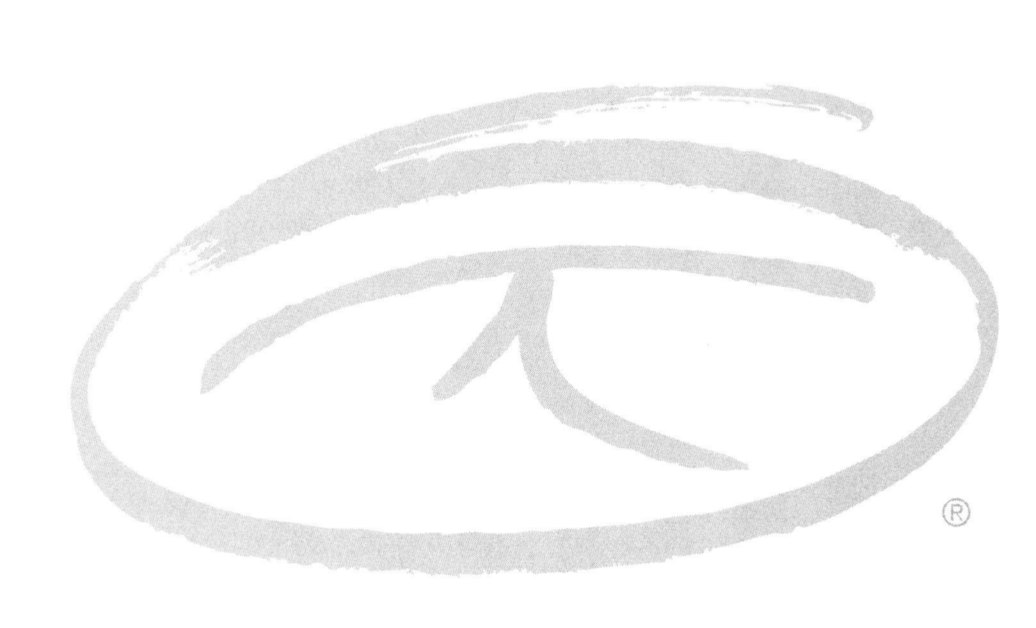

Index

Zero Balancing and . . .

Welcome

to the Zero Balancing Health Association

When you study with International Alliance of Healthcare Educators (IAHE) you gain a lifelong resource for exceptional continuing education and professional support. With every course you take you can be assured of our commitment to provide you with the highest level of instruction and service possible in the classroom and beyond.

IAHE benefits include:

- Curriculums designed by the modality developer or top leaders in their field
- Classes taught by practicing healthcare professionals who have completed extensive teaching apprenticeship programs
- Seminars designed to enable you to confidently begin utilizing what you have learned with clients
- Contact hours to satisfy many cases of continuing-education unit (CEU) requirements
- Certificate of Attendance and CEU letter provided on the last day of class
- Networking with colleagues in class and beyond—class roster access e-mailed to you within a few weeks following class
- Certification programs valued and recognized worldwide
- Reduced tuition for course review
- Workshops in more than 400 cities and 60 countries
- Access to study groups
- Personal online account for accessing transaction receipts
- Skilled educational-services counselors to assist you in registering for workshops, selecting products and providing general information
- Access to a wide array of support material containing valuable insights into new research, techniques and best practices
- Free membership through the International Association of Healthcare Practitioners (IAHP)
- Eligibility to upgrade to IAHP Medallion Membership, with benefits that include access to online class review material, enhanced listing status on iahp.com, a customized online therapist profile, and unlimited access to rosters of classes you've attended

We look forward to seeing you at a seminar—an exceptional learning and professional development experience.

IAHE.com

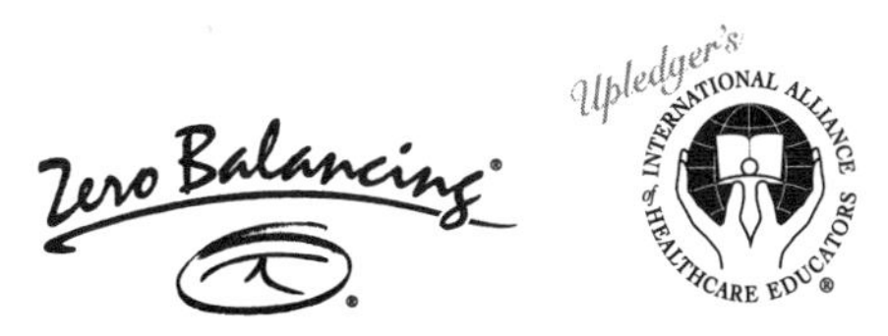

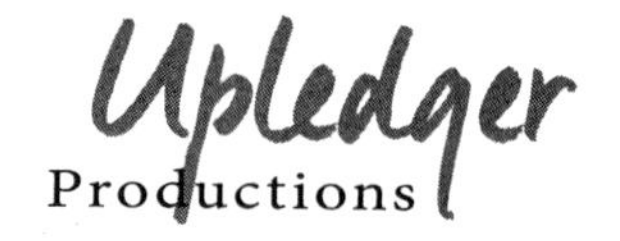

Your source for educational excellence.

Titles also available:

The Alchemy of Touch–Moving Towards Mastery through the Lens of Zero Balancing

An Answer to Your Pain

CranioSacral Therapy for Health and Healing

CranioSacral Therapy: Touchstone for Natural Healing

The Deep Massage Book–How to Combine Structure and Energy in Bodywork

Inner Bridges–A Guide to Energy Movement and Body Structure

SomatoEmotional Release: Deciphering the Language of Life

Your Inner Physician and You

Zero Balancing Expanded: The Attitude of Awaiting a Fish

www.Upledger.com

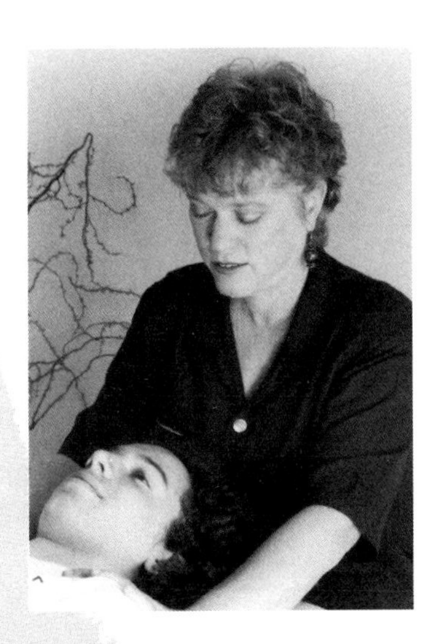

Zero Balancing Health Association
Columbia, MD
410.381.8956 phone
410.381.9634 fax
zbha@zerobalancing.com

www.zerobalancing.com
www.youtube.com/user/zerobalancing
www.facebook.com/ZBNorthAmerica
@zerobalancing
Zero Balancing North America

Veronica Quarry, MS, MSPT
Certified Zero Balancing and
CranioSacral Therapist
617 480-3648

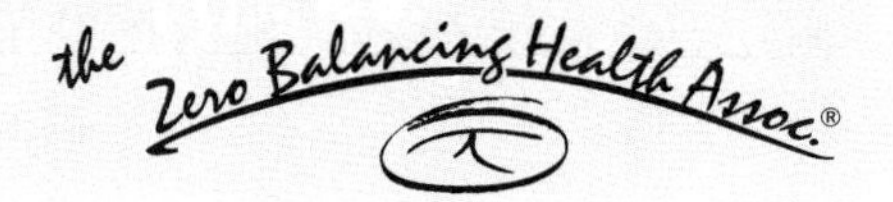

Zero Balancing®

Bridging the Mind and Body Through Touch

"Experience has shown that people's lives feel smoother when they're getting regular body-mind therapy; it is an avenue toward discovering your true nature."

Fritz Frederick Smith, M.D.

the Zero Balancing Health Assoc.®